Quick and Easy Anti-Inflammatory Fibromyalgia Cookbook

Nutritious and Delicious Gut-Friendly Recipes for Management and Treatment of Fibro Symptoms and Effective Nutrients Absorption

Alice L. Jordan

1

Copyright © 2024 by Alice L. Jordan

Table of Contents

Introduction

In the summer of last year, the fluorescent lights of the community center, buzzed overhead, casting a sterile glow on the sea of faces staring back at us, We, a compassionate team of nutritionists and dietitians, were on a mission – to educate a room full of people wrestling with the invisible monster known as fibromyalgia, fatigue, pain, sleep disturbances, – these were the unwelcome companions most carried with them. We were also there to educate the caregivers and the loved ones of those living with fibromyalgia on the best practices with anti-inflammatory foods. My heart ached for their struggle, a feeling I knew all too well from countless patient interactions.

Our arsenal? Not scalpels or medications, but colorful flyers and well-worn pamphlets. We talked about the magic of anti-inflammatory foods, the warriors on our plates that could fight the silent battle within. We shared recipes that were as delicious as they were good for you, meals that wouldn't sap their already limited energy. We spoke of turmeric's golden power, the calming whispers of chamomile tea, the vibrant antioxidants in berries.

The room, once quiet with resignation, crackled with a newfound spark. Hope flickered in their eyes as they flipped through the pamphlets, highlighting recipes and scribbling notes. We weren't promising a cure, but a chance to take back some control, a chance to find pockets of relief in a world often painted with pain.

The weeks that followed were a whirlwind. Our phones rang off the hook with calls from people eager to share their experiences. Emails flooded our inboxes, each message carrying a weight of gratitude that left me choked with emotion. There was Sarah, who finally managed a full night's sleep for the first time in years. John, whose chronic bloating had subsided, allowing him to enjoy a simple meal with his family. And Mary, who wrote about the newfound energy that allowed her to take a walk in the park again, the sun warm on her face.

These weren't just words on a page; they were testaments to the power of food, the transformative potential hidden within a simple plate. Their stories fueled a fire within me, a burning desire to share this knowledge with a wider audience. This book, my friends, is the culmination of that desire. It's a roadmap to navigate the world of anti-inflammatory eating for those living with fibromyalgia. It's a battle cry, a call to arms against the limitations the disease tries to impose.

Within these pages, you'll find not just recipes but strategies. We'll delve into the science of anti-inflammatory foods, but more importantly, we'll translate that science into simple, actionable steps. You'll discover meal plans that fit your busy schedule, tips for grocery shopping, and even tricks to navigate social gatherings without sacrificing your dietary needs.

This journey won't be easy. There will be days when fatigue wins, and reaching for comfort food seems easier. But remember, you're not alone. You have this book, a companion on your path to a better tomorrow. You have the countless stories of others who have found relief through food. And most importantly, you have the unwavering strength within you, the same strength that brought you here.

So, turn the page, my friend. Let's rewrite the narrative of fibromyalgia together, one delicious bite at a time. Let's reclaim your well-being, your energy, your life.

Understanding Fibromyalgia

Fibromyalgia can feel like a bit of a mystery. It's a condition that causes widespread pain and tenderness throughout your body, along with fatigue that can leave you feeling wiped out. Sleep often becomes a battleground, with restless nights and waking up feeling unrested. On top of that, many people with fibromyalgia experience things like brain fog (trouble concentrating), headaches, and even mood swings. It's a lot to handle, and it can definitely make everyday life challenging.

Fighting Fibromyalgia with Anti-Inflammatory Diets

While there isn't a known cure for fibromyalgia, there are ways to manage your symptoms and feel better. One powerful tool you can use in this fight against fibromyalgia is your diet.
Research suggests that anti-inflammatory foods can be a game-changer. These are foods rich in nutrients that can help reduce inflammation in your body, which may be a contributing factor to fibromyalgia pain.

By incorporating more anti-inflammatory foods into your meals, you might experience:

- **Reduced pain:** These foods can help calm down the internal fire that contributes to fibromyalgia pain.
- **Improved sleep:** Certain anti-inflammatory foods can promote better sleep quality, leaving you feeling more rested.

- **Increased energy:** By managing inflammation, you might have more energy to tackle your day.
- **Overall better well-being:** Eating a diet rich in anti-inflammatory foods can contribute to a healthier you, both physically and mentally.

Unveiling the Inflammatory Link in Fibromyalgia

Fibromyalgia presents a unique challenge for many patients. The widespread pain, fatigue, and sleep disruptions can significantly impact quality of life. While the exact cause remains under investigation, recent research highlights a potential cause: chronic, low-grade inflammation.

Think of inflammation as the body's internal alarm system. When triggered by injury or infection, it sends white blood cells – our body's firefighters – to the scene. This acute inflammation is a vital healing process. However, in some cases, this response becomes dysregulated, leading to chronic inflammation.

In the context of fibromyalgia, medical practitioners suspect this low-grade, persistent inflammation may be contributing to your pain and other symptoms. It's not a full-blown fire, but more like a simmering ember that disrupts various bodily processes.

The exciting news is that dietary interventions can play a significant role in managing inflammation. Certain foods act as natural anti-inflammatory agents, potentially offering relief for your fibromyalgia symptoms.

Anti-Inflammatory Food as Medicine for Fibromyalgia

Now that we've shed light on the potential role of inflammation in fibromyalgia, let's introduce the anti-inflammatory foods. These powerhouses are packed with nutrients that can help your body fight off that persistent, low-grade inflammation, potentially leading to significant improvements in your overall well-being.

Think of these foods as natural firefighters. They contain compounds that can help:

- **Reduce inflammation:** Certain nutrients like omega-3 fatty acids and antioxidants work to calm the internal fire that contributes to fibromyalgia pain.
- **Boost your immune system:** A healthy immune system helps your body fight off infections and prevents unnecessary inflammation. Anti-inflammatory foods often come loaded with vitamins, minerals, and antioxidants that support your immune function.
- **Promote gut health:** A healthy gut microbiome plays a crucial role in overall inflammation. Some anti-inflammatory foods, like those rich in prebiotics and probiotics, can help nourish the good gut bacteria, promoting a balanced gut environment.

The benefits of incorporating anti-inflammatory foods into your diet for fibromyalgia management can be multifaceted. You might experience:

- **Reduced pain and stiffness:** By calming inflammation, these foods can potentially help lessen the widespread pain and stiffness associated with fibromyalgia.
- **Improved energy levels:** Chronic inflammation can zap your energy. Anti-inflammatory foods may help by supporting your body's natural processes and reducing fatigue.

- **Enhanced sleep quality:** Certain anti-inflammatory foods can promote better sleep, allowing you to wake up feeling more rested and refreshed.
- **Overall better well-being:** By managing inflammation and supporting your immune system, anti-inflammatory foods can contribute to a healthier you, both physically and mentally.

Chapter 1: Building Your Anti-Inflammatory Kitchen

Essential Pantry Staples

Conquering fibromyalgia with delicious, anti-inflammatory meals starts with a well-equipped pantry. Here's your essential shopping list, categorized for easy reference:

Healthy Fats

- **Extra Virgin Olive Oil:** Use it for drizzling, sauteing, salad dressings, and even baking.
- **Avocado Oil:** A heart-healthy alternative for high-heat cooking like searing or stir-frying.
- **Nuts & Seeds:** Stock up on raw or dry-roasted options like almonds, walnuts, chia seeds, and flaxseeds. Sprinkle them on salads, yogurt, or oatmeal, or enjoy them as a healthy snack.

Spices

- **Turmeric:** Use it in curries, soups, roasted vegetables, or even golden milk lattes.
- **Ginger:** This pungent root offers anti-inflammatory and pain-relieving properties. Enjoy it fresh in stir-fries or teas, or in its ground form for baked goods or curries.
- **Garlic:** A delicious and versatile herb with well-documented anti-inflammatory benefits. Use it fresh or dried in a variety of dishes.

- **Black Pepper:** Not just for taste, black pepper also enhances the absorption of curcumin from turmeric, making them a powerful anti-inflammatory duo. Grind it fresh for maximum flavor.
- **Cinnamon:** This warm spice boasts anti-inflammatory properties and adds sweetness to dishes without refined sugar. Perfect for oatmeal, curries, or even a sprinkle on roasted vegetables.

Pantry Powerhouses

- **Dried Beans & Lentils:** Budget-friendly and packed with protein and fiber, these are anti-inflammatory stars. They're perfect for soups, stews, salads, and even dips.
- **Canned Tomatoes:** A versatile pantry staple for quick and easy meals. Choose diced, crushed, or whole peeled tomatoes depending on your recipe. Opt for BPA-free cans whenever possible.
- **Low-Sodium Vegetable Broth:** Use this flavorful base for soups, stews, or to add depth to sauces. Choose a low-sodium option to control your daily salt intake.
- **Apple Cider Vinegar:** This vinegar has potential anti-inflammatory properties and adds a tangy flavor to salad dressings and marinades.
- **Fresh Herbs:** Consider keeping fresh herbs like parsley, cilantro, or basil on hand for adding a burst of flavor and essential nutrients to your dishes. They're perfect for garnishes, salads, or infused in olive oil.

Keep the following Anti-Inflammatory powerhouse fresh in the fridge. Your refrigerator will be your anti-inflammatory ally, stocked with vibrant fruits, vegetables, and lean protein sources like:

Fruits

- **Berries:** These antioxidant powerhouses are loaded with anti-inflammatory properties. Stock up on blueberries, strawberries, raspberries, and cherries.
- **Citrus Fruits:** Rich in vitamin C, oranges, grapefruits, and grapefruits offer a refreshing and anti-inflammatory boost.
- **Pineapples:** This tropical treat contains bromelain, an enzyme with potential anti-inflammatory benefits.
- **Melons:** Watermelon and cantaloupe are packed with hydrating water and antioxidants, contributing to overall well-being.

Vegetables

- **Leafy Greens:** Kale, spinach, Swiss chard, and collard greens are all anti-inflammatory champions. They're perfect for salads, smoothies, or sauteed as a side dish.
- **Cruciferous Vegetables:** Broccoli, cauliflower, Brussels sprouts, and bok choy are loaded with sulforaphane, a compound with anti-inflammatory properties.
- **Bell Peppers:** Available in various colors, bell peppers are rich in antioxidants and vitamin C, supporting a healthy inflammatory response.
- **Avocados:** These creamy fruits (yes, they're fruits!) are a healthy fat powerhouse. Enjoy them sliced on toast, in salads, or mashed into guacamole.

Lean Protein Sources

- **Fatty Fish:** Salmon, tuna, sardines, and mackerel are rich in omega-3 fatty acids, known for their anti-inflammatory benefits. Aim for 2-3 servings per week.
- **Chicken & Turkey Breast:** Lean protein sources like chicken and turkey breast are perfect for grilling, baking, or adding to salads.
- **Eggs:** A budget-friendly and versatile protein source, eggs are also a good source of choline, which may play a role in reducing inflammation.

While most fruits and vegetables benefit from the cool crispness of the fridge, some are better stored at room temperature. Store the following Anti-Inflammatory ingredients under room temperature:

- **Tomatoes:** Chilling tomatoes can dull their flavor and texture. Keep them on your counter at room temperature.
- **Stone Fruits:** Peaches, nectarines, plums, and apricots ripen best at room temperature. Once ripe, you can store them in the fridge for a few days.
- **Bananas:** Cold temperatures can turn banana peels brown and the flesh mushy. Store them at room temperature and refrigerate only if they become overly ripe.
- **Avocados:** Never store unripe avocados in the fridge. Let them ripen at room temperature, then refrigerate once they're soft.

Smart Shopping Tips

Living with fibromyalgia can make even simple tasks like grocery shopping feel overwhelming. Fatigue, pain, and a lack of motivation can leave you wanting to skip the store altogether. Here are some smart shopping tips to make grocery shopping a breeze, freeing up your energy for the things that truly matter:

Plan Like a Pro

- **Meal Planning is Your Ally:** Before venturing out, plan your meals for the week. This minimizes impulse buys and ensures you have everything on hand to cook healthy, anti-inflammatory meals. There are plenty of online meal planning resources or apps that can help you streamline the process. And included in this book is a comprehensive anti-inflammatory meal plan.
- **Embrace Online Ordering and Delivery:** Take advantage of online grocery shopping and delivery services. This allows you to browse from the comfort of your couch, build your cart, and have groceries delivered right to your doorstep.
- **Make a List (and Check it Twice):** Create a detailed shopping list to avoid unnecessary browsing and impulse purchases. Group similar items together to optimize your route through the store.

Shop Smart, Not Hard

- **Befriend the Freezer:** Stock up on frozen fruits and vegetables. They're flash-frozen at peak ripeness, retaining nutrients and offering a convenient, pre-washed option. Opt for frozen options without added sugars or sauces.
- **Embrace Canned Goods:** Canned beans, lentils, and tomatoes are shelf-stable, budget-friendly, and perfect for quick meals. Choose low-sodium versions to control your salt intake.

- **Pre-Cut is Your Friend:** Consider buying pre-cut vegetables like broccoli florets, baby carrots, or bagged salad mixes. This saves precious time and energy when you're feeling wiped out.
- **Batch Cooking is Your Superpower:** When you have a good energy day, consider batch cooking a few meals in advance. Divide them into portions and freeze them for those days when cooking seems like a distant dream.

Delivery Services Can Be Lifesavers

- **Meal Kit Delivery Services:** Explore meal kit delivery services that portion and pre-prep ingredients for delicious, healthy meals. This minimizes prep time and allows you to cook delicious, anti-inflammatory meals without the hassle.
- **Grocery Delivery Services:** Many grocery stores offer delivery services where you can order online and choose a delivery slot that fits your schedule. This eliminates the need to navigate crowded stores, saving you precious energy.

Bonus Tip: If you do venture out to the store

- **Utilize Store Amenities:** Many stores offer electric carts or scooter rentals. Don't hesitate to use them to help you navigate the aisles and minimize fatigue.
- **Dress for Comfort:** Wear comfortable clothing and shoes that can support you while you shop.

Reading Food Labels and Spotting Sneaky Inflammatory Ingredients

Living with fibromyalgia makes you become a detective in your own kitchen. Now, get equipped with the skills to decode food labels and identify sneaky inflammatory ingredients that might be hiding in plain sight. Here's what to watch out for:

- **Added Sugars:** Excessive sugar intake can contribute to inflammation. Be on the lookout for these hidden sugar sources:
- **Look Beyond "Sugar":** Check for ingredients like "high fructose corn syrup," "cane sugar," "brown sugar," "honey," or "maple syrup." These all contribute to added sugars.
- **Beware of Disguises:** Watch out for ingredients ending in "-ose," like sucrose, maltose, or dextrose – they're all forms of added sugar.
- **The Power of Numbers:** Scan the "Nutrition Facts" label. Aim for products with low added sugars. Ideally, they should be below 10 grams per serving, and the closer to zero, the better.

Unhealthy Fats

Not all fats are created equal. While some fats are essential for good health, others can promote inflammation. Here's what to avoid:

- **Trans Fats:** These are the worst offenders. Thankfully, trans fats are largely banned in the US. However, it's still wise to check the label and avoid anything with "partially hydrogenated oils."
- **Saturated Fats:** Limit saturated fats, often found in high quantities in animal products like fatty cuts of meat, processed meats, and full-fat dairy products.

- **Beware of Hidden Saturated Fats:** Saturated fats can lurk in unexpected places like baked goods, fried foods, and commercially prepared snacks.

Other Inflammatory Ingredients

While added sugars and unhealthy fats are top priorities, keep an eye out for these as well:

- **Refined Grains:** White bread, pasta, and white rice can contribute to inflammation. Opt for whole grains like brown rice, quinoa, or whole-wheat bread whenever possible.
- **Omega-6 Fatty Acids:** While omega-3 fatty acids are anti-inflammatory, excessive omega-6 intake can be pro-inflammatory. Be mindful of vegetable oils high in omega-6, like corn oil and soybean oil.

Kitchen Essentials for Quick and Easy meal Prep

Here are some essential tools to streamline your anti-inflammatory meal prep and free up your energy for the things that matter:

Chopping Essentials

- **Sharp Knives:** A good quality chef's knife and a paring knife are your chopping companions-in-arms. Invest in sharp knives – they'll make prepping vegetables and fruits quicker and easier, minimizing stress on your joints.
- **Cutting Boards:** Choose a sturdy cutting board that protects your countertops and is easy on your wrists. Consider different sizes for various tasks.

Cooking Essentials

- **Sheet Pans:** These versatile pans are perfect for roasting vegetables, baking fish, or even prepping one-pan meals. Toss your ingredients together, throw them in the oven, and enjoy a delicious, healthy meal with minimal cleanup.
- **Slow Cooker:** A slow cooker is a lifesaver for busy days. Throw in your ingredients in the morning, and come home to a hot, home-cooked meal ready to enjoy. Perfect for soups, stews, and braised meats.
- **Blender/Food Processor:** These countertop companions can be your allies in quick meal prep. Use them to whip up smoothies, healthy dips, salad dressings, or grind nuts and seeds.

Storage Essentials

- **Airtight Containers:** Store prepared vegetables, cooked leftovers, or portioned snacks in airtight containers. This keeps them fresh, prevents spoilage, and allows for easy grab-and-go options throughout the week.
- **Silicone Molds:** Portion out yogurt parfaits, freeze smoothie cubes, or bake healthy muffins – silicone molds offer endless possibilities for healthy meal prep and portion control.

Bonus Tools

- **Spiralizer:** This handy gadget turns vegetables like zucchini or sweet potatoes into noodles, creating a fun and healthy alternative to traditional pasta dishes.

- **Rice Cooker:** A perfect tool for cooking fluffy rice, quinoa, or brown rice – all staples for anti-inflammatory meals.

Remember that you don't need to go overboard and buy every kitchen gadget out there. Start with a few key pieces that suit your cooking style and budget. As you explore the recipes in this book, you'll discover which tools become your go-to favorites for creating delicious and nutritious anti-inflammatory meals.

Chapter 2: Understanding Anti-Inflammatory Ingredients

Fruits (berries, cherries, citrus)

Fruits are nature's candy, and for those managing fibromyalgia, these vibrant options offer a delicious and anti-inflammatory punch:

Berries and Their Benefits

- **Berries (blueberries, strawberries, raspberries):** These little gems are packed with antioxidants called anthocyanins, which have powerful anti-inflammatory properties. Studies suggest anthocyanins may help reduce pain and inflammation throughout the body, potentially offering relief for fibromyalgia symptoms.
- **Bonus:** Berries are also a good source of fiber, which can help with gut health and overall well-being.

Cherry and Their Benefits

- **Cherries:** Don't underestimate the power of these ruby-red fruits. Cherries are rich in compounds called anthocyanins (similar to those in berries) and unique antioxidants called proanthocyanidins. These work together to reduce inflammation and may even offer some pain-relieving properties.

Citrus and Their Benefits

- **Citrus fruits (oranges, grapefruits, grapefruits):** Packed with vitamin C, these sunshine-colored fruits are well-known for their immune-boosting properties. Vitamin C is also an antioxidant that can help fight inflammation in the body.

Here's how incorporating these fruits into your diet can benefit you:

- **Reduced Pain and Stiffness:** The anti-inflammatory properties of these fruits may help lessen the widespread pain and stiffness associated with fibromyalgia.
- **Improved Energy Levels:** Chronic inflammation can zap your energy. By managing inflammation, these fruits may help you feel more energetic throughout the day.
- **Overall Well-being:** The antioxidants and vitamins in these fruits contribute to a healthy immune system and overall well-being, which is crucial for managing fibromyalgia.

Tips for Enjoying these Anti-inflammatory Fruits:

- **Snack on them fresh:** Enjoy them as a mid-morning or afternoon snack, or add them to yogurt parfaits.
- **Blend them into smoothies:** Make a refreshing and anti-inflammatory smoothie by blending berries, cherries, or citrus fruits with yogurt, spinach, and a splash of water or plant-based milk.

- **Bake with them:** Add a burst of flavor and antioxidants to muffins, pancakes, or even savory dishes like chicken salad.

Vegetables (leafy greens, cruciferous vegetables, tomatoes)

When it comes to fighting inflammation with food, vegetables are your champions. Let's explore the powerhouses you mentioned and how they can benefit people with fibromyalgia:

Leafy Green Goodness

- **Kale, spinach, Swiss chard, collard greens:** These dark, leafy greens are overflowing with nutrients and anti-inflammatory compounds. They're rich in antioxidants like beta-carotene and vitamin K, which can help reduce inflammation and oxidative stress in the body.

Cruciferous Crusaders

- **Broccoli, cauliflower, Brussels sprouts, bok choy:** These cruciferous vegetables are loaded with sulforaphane, a powerful compound with well-documented anti-inflammatory properties. Studies suggest sulforaphane may help modulate the immune system's response to inflammation, potentially offering relief for fibromyalgia symptoms.

Tomatoes

- **Tomatoes:** While not technically a green veggie, tomatoes deserve a mention! They're a source of lycopene, an antioxidant with anti-inflammatory properties. While research is ongoing, some studies suggest lycopene may help reduce inflammation and improve overall well-being.

How these Veggies can Benefit Fibromyalgia

- **Reduced Pain and Inflammation:** The anti-inflammatory properties of these vegetables may help manage the widespread pain and inflammation associated with fibromyalgia.
- **Improved Gut Health:** Leafy greens and cruciferous vegetables are rich in fiber, which promotes a healthy gut microbiome. A healthy gut is linked to reduced inflammation throughout the body.
- **Enhanced Nutrient Intake:** These vegetables are packed with essential vitamins, minerals, and antioxidants that contribute to overall well-being and a healthy immune system, both important for managing fibromyalgia.

Tips for Savoring these Anti-inflammatory Veggies

- **Salads are your canvas:** Enjoy them fresh in salads with a light vinaigrette dressing.
- **Roast them for a twist:** Roasting vegetables brings out their natural sweetness. Toss them with olive oil, spices, and roast for a delicious side dish.
- **Sneak them in:** Add chopped leafy greens to smoothies, soups, or even omelets.

- **Tomatoes add versatility:** Enjoy them sliced in salads, blended into gazpacho, or cooked into tomato sauce for a healthy pasta dish.

Lean Protein Sources (fish, poultry, beans)

Choosing the right protein sources is crucial for managing fibromyalgia. Here's how these options can be anti-inflammatory allies:

Fish

- **Fatty Fish (salmon, tuna, sardines, mackerel):** These champions are brimming with omega-3 fatty acids, particularly EPA and DHA. These polyunsaturated fats have well-documented anti-inflammatory properties and may help reduce pain and stiffness associated with fibromyalgia. Aim for 2-3 servings of fatty fish per week.

Poultry

- **Chicken & Turkey Breast:** Lean protein sources like chicken and turkey breast are excellent alternatives to red meat. They offer essential protein for muscle building and repair, without the saturated fat that can contribute to inflammation.

Beans

- **Beans (black beans, kidney beans, chickpeas, lentils):** Don't underestimate the power of these humble legumes. Beans are a plant-based protein source rich in fiber and antioxidants. They can also help regulate blood sugar, which can indirectly contribute to better pain management.

Their Benefits for Fibromyalgia Management

- **Reduced Inflammation:** Omega-3 fatty acids in fish and the anti-inflammatory properties of beans can help manage inflammation, potentially leading to less pain and stiffness.
- **Improved Muscle Function:** Protein is essential for muscle health. Lean protein sources can help maintain muscle strength and function, which can be impacted by fibromyalgia.
- **Aid Satiety:** Protein is well known to make you feel fuller for longer. This can help regulate blood sugar and potentially reduce fatigue, a common symptom of fibromyalgia.

Tips on How to Include these Lean Protein Sources

- **Bake or grill your fish:** Simple cooking methods like baking or grilling help preserve the omega-3 content in fish.
- **Get creative with poultry:** Chicken and turkey breasts can be versatile ingredients. Experiment with different herbs, spices, and marinades to create flavorful dishes.
- **Explore the bean world:** Beans are incredibly versatile. Enjoy them in soups, stews, salads, dips, or even veggie burgers.
- **Combine protein and fiber:** Pair your lean protein sources with whole grains or vegetables for a balanced and satisfying meal.

Healthy Fats (olive oil, avocado, nuts and seeds)

Fat isn't the enemy. In fact, certain healthy fats play a crucial role in managing fibromyalgia. Here's how these healthy fats can benefit you:

Olive Oil: A Mediterranean Marvel

- **Extra Virgin Olive Oil:** This liquid gold is packed with monounsaturated fats, particularly oleic acid. Studies suggest oleic acid may have anti-inflammatory properties and can help reduce pain and improve function in people with chronic inflammatory conditions. Drizzle it on salads, use it for sauteing, or enjoy it in a simple dipping sauce with balsamic vinegar.

Avocado

- **Avocados:** These heart-healthy fruits are a rich source of healthy fats, specifically monounsaturated fats and some omega-3s. The fats in avocados may contribute to an anti-inflammatory response in the body. Enjoy them mashed on toast, sliced in salads, or blended into a delicious guacamole.

Nuts & Seeds

- **Nuts (almonds, walnuts, chia seeds, flaxseeds):** Don't underestimate these little nutritional powerhouses. Nuts and seeds are rich in healthy fats, including monounsaturated fats, omega-3s, and fiber. These fats, along with other nutrients in nuts and seeds, may help reduce inflammation and contribute to overall well-being. Enjoy them as a snack, sprinkle them on salads or yogurt, or use them in homemade granola bars.

Their Benefits for Fibromyalgia Management

- **Reduced Inflammation:** The healthy fats in these foods offer anti-inflammatory properties, potentially leading to less pain and stiffness.
- **Improved Satiety:** Healthy fats can help you feel fuller for longer, which can regulate blood sugar and potentially reduce fatigue, a common symptom of fibromyalgia.
- **Enhanced Nutrient Intake:** These foods are packed with essential vitamins, minerals, and antioxidants that contribute to overall well-being, which is crucial for managing fibromyalgia.

Tips for Including these Healthy Fats

- **Incorporate them daily:** Aim to include a healthy fat source at most meals and snacks.
- **Variety is key:** Explore different types of nuts and seeds to keep your taste buds happy.
- **Moderation matters:** While healthy, nuts and seeds are calorie-dense. So it's highly advisable to consume them in moderation as part of a balanced diet.

Spices and Herbs (turmeric, ginger, garlic, etc.)

When it comes to managing fibromyalgia, don't underestimate the power of your spice rack. These flavorful additions enhance your dishes and also offer some impressive anti-inflammatory benefits. Here are some highly recommended anti-inflammatory spices and herbs to consider:

- **Turmeric:** This vibrant yellow spice boasts a powerful anti-inflammatory compound called curcumin. Studies suggest curcumin may help reduce pain and inflammation, potentially offering relief for fibromyalgia symptoms. Enjoy turmeric in curries, soups, roasted vegetables, or even a golden milk latte.

- **Ginger:** This pungent root offers anti-inflammatory and pain-relieving properties. Ginger may help reduce muscle pain and inflammation, potentially offering some relief for fibromyalgia symptoms. Enjoy it fresh in stir-fries or teas, or in its ground form for baked goods or curries.
- **Garlic:** A delicious and versatile herb, garlic also has well-documented anti-inflammatory benefits. Studies suggest garlic may help reduce inflammation and improve overall heart health. Use it fresh or dried in a variety of dishes.
- **Black Pepper:** This ingredient is not just for adding flavor. Black pepper enhances the absorption of curcumin from turmeric, making them a powerful anti-inflammatory duo. Grind it fresh for maximum flavor.
- **Cinnamon:** This warm spice boasts anti-inflammatory properties and adds sweetness to dishes without refined sugar. Perfect for oatmeal, curries, or even a sprinkle on roasted vegetables.
- **Cayenne pepper:** This pepper contains capsaicin, which may help reduce pain perception.
- **Cloves:** Cloves offer anti-inflammatory properties and a unique flavor.
- **Rosemary:** Rosemary may help improve circulation and has antioxidant properties.

Their Benefits for Fibromyalgia Management

- **Reduced Inflammation:** The anti-inflammatory properties of these spices and herbs may help manage inflammation, potentially leading to less pain and stiffness.
- **Improved Flavor:** The fact is, bland food is boring. Spices and herbs add exciting flavors to your meals, making healthy eating more enjoyable.

Tips for Using Spices and Herbs
- **Experiment:** Don't be afraid to try different spices and herbs to discover flavor combinations you enjoy.
- **Fresh or dried:** Both fresh and dried spices and herbs offer benefits. Fresh herbs tend to have a more vibrant flavor, while dried spices are convenient and have a longer shelf life.
- **Whisk them in:** Add spices and herbs during cooking to allow their flavors to develop.

How to Incorporate Anti-inflammatory Ingredients into Your Daily Meals

Incorporating anti-inflammatory ingredients into your daily meals is a powerful tool you can use to manage symptoms and improve your health. Here's how to create a delicious and functional anti-inflammatory meal plan:

Start Your Day with a Powerful Punch

Breakfast: Aim for a balanced meal with protein, healthy fats, and anti-inflammatory powerhouses.

- **Option 1:** Greek yogurt with berries, walnuts, and a sprinkle of chia seeds.
- **Option 2:** Scrambled eggs with chopped spinach, tomatoes, and a slice of whole-wheat toast drizzled with olive oil.
- **Option 3:** A smoothie packed with spinach, banana, almond milk, and a scoop of protein powder.

Lunchtime: Focus on variety and nutrient density.
- **Option 1:** A colorful salad with grilled salmon, quinoa, roasted vegetables, and a lemon-herb dressing.
- **Option 2:** Lentil soup with a whole-grain roll and a side salad.
- **Option 3:** Turkey breast sandwich on whole-wheat bread with avocado, lettuce, tomato, and a drizzle of olive oil.

Dinner: Dinner is the time to get creative and explore different flavors.
- **Option 1:** Baked salmon with roasted Brussels sprouts and sweet potato wedges, seasoned with turmeric and rosemary.
- **Option 2:** Chicken stir-fry with brown rice, colorful vegetables, and a ginger-garlic sauce.
- **Option 3:** Vegetarian chili packed with beans, vegetables, and spices like cumin and chili powder.

Don't Forget Snacks: Snacking strategically helps regulate blood sugar and keeps you fueled throughout the day.
- **Option 1:** Apple slices with almond butter.
- **Option 2:** Carrot sticks with hummus.
- **Option 3:** Handful of mixed nuts and berries.

Remember, these are just examples, so be creative and experiment with different ingredients based on your preferences and dietary needs.

Bonus meal prep tips
- **Read food labels:** Be mindful of added sugars, unhealthy fats, and hidden inflammatory ingredients as earlier discussed above.
- **Cook in bulk:** When you have good energy days, consider preparing meals in advance to save time and energy.
- **Stay hydrated:** Drinking plenty of water is crucial for overall health and can help manage fatigue.

Beyond meal prep and food, lifestyle modifications is also crucial for managing fibromyalgia by adopting the following:
- **Manage stress:** Stress can worsen fibromyalgia symptoms. Relaxation techniques like deep breathing, yoga, or meditation can help in management of stress.
- **Prioritize sleep:** When possible, ensure you get up to seven to eight hours of quality sleep each night.
- **Gentle exercise:** Regular physical activity, even low-impact exercises like walking or swimming, can improve pain and flexibility.

It's also important for you to always consult your doctor or a registered dietitian for personalized guidance on managing your fibromyalgia with diet and lifestyle modifications.

Substitution Ideas for Dietary Restrictions (vegetarian, vegan, gluten-free)

Dietary restrictions don't have to limit your access to delicious and anti-inflammatory meals. Here are some substitution options for vegetarians, vegans, and those with gluten sensitivity:

Vegetarian & Vegan Swaps

- **Protein Power:** Instead of fish or chicken, explore vegetarian and vegan protein sources like:
- **Beans & Lentils:** These powerhouses are packed with protein and fiber, making them excellent choices for building a hearty and anti-inflammatory meal.
- **Tofu & Tempeh:** These soy-based options offer a meaty texture and are great sources of plant-based protein.
- **Eggs:** For vegetarians, eggs are a complete protein source and a good source of choline, which may play a role in reducing inflammation.
- **Nuts & Seeds:** While not a complete protein source on their own, incorporating nuts and seeds into your diet adds protein, healthy fats, and fiber.

Dairy Alternatives

For those with dairy sensitivities, there are many delicious plant-based alternatives available

- **Milk:** Choose from a variety of plant-based milks like almond milk, soy milk, oat milk, or coconut milk. Opt for unsweetened versions whenever possible.

- **Yogurt:** Look for coconut yogurt, soy yogurt, or almond yogurt – all great options for incorporating probiotics and maintaining a healthy gut microbiome.
- **Cheese:** Explore dairy-free cheese alternatives made from cashews, almonds, or soy.

Gluten-Free Twists

Swap out wheat-based ingredients for delicious gluten-free alternatives:
- **Breads & Grains:** Explore options like gluten-free bread made with almond flour, coconut flour, or brown rice flour. You can also use quinoa, brown rice, or buckwheat as grain alternatives.
- **Pasta:** There's a wide variety of gluten-free pasta options available, including those made from chickpea flour, lentil flour, or brown rice.

Here are some specific meal examples incorporating these substitutions:
- **Vegetarian Breakfast:** Whole-wheat toast (or gluten-free alternative) topped with mashed avocado, a fried egg, and sliced tomato.
- **Vegan Lunch:** Quinoa bowl with roasted vegetables, black beans, a dollop of guacamole, and a lemon-tahini dressing.
- **Gluten-Free Dinner:** Baked cod with roasted sweet potato fries and steamed broccoli drizzled with olive oil and a sprinkle of paprika.

These are just a few ideas – get creative and explore the vast world of vegetarian, vegan, and gluten-free recipes. Experiment with different ingredients and flavors to find what works best for your taste buds and dietary needs.

Chapter 3: Quick and Easy Anti-Inflammatory Meals

Importance of Meal Planning for Managing Fibromyalgia

Meal planning isn't just about convenience — it's a powerful tool for managing symptoms, saving time and energy. Here's why meal planning is a game-changer:

- **Reduced Decision Fatigue:** Fibromyalgia can leave you feeling drained. Planning your meals in advance eliminates the daily struggle of "what to eat?" This helps you reserve mental energy for other chores or simply allows you to relax.
- **Control Over Ingredients:** By planning your meals, you're in control of what goes into your plate. You can choose anti-inflammatory ingredients, eliminate processed foods, and tailor your meals to any dietary restrictions you may have.
- **Minimizes Painful Flare-Ups:** Skipping meals or relying on convenience foods can lead to blood sugar fluctuations, which can contribute to fatigue and pain flares. Meal planning ensures you're eating regular, balanced meals that keep your blood sugar stable.
- **Saves Time and Energy:** No more last-minute grocery runs or scrambling to figure out dinner after a long day. Meal planning allows you to shop efficiently and cook in bulk on good energy days, saving precious time and energy throughout the week.

- **Reduces Stress:** The uncertainty of "what to eat" can be stressful. Meal planning eliminates this stressor, allowing you to focus on other aspects of managing fibromyalgia and living your life.

- **Promotes Healthy Eating Habits:** Meal planning encourages you to focus on incorporating a variety of anti-inflammatory ingredients like fruits, vegetables, lean protein sources, and healthy fats. This promotes long-term health benefits.

- **Boosts Energy Levels:** Eating balanced, regular meals helps regulate blood sugar, which can combat fatigue and enhance increased energy throughout the day.

- **Empowerment and Confidence:** Taking control of your meals is an empowering act. You're making conscious choices about your health and well-being, which can boost confidence and self-esteem in managing your fibromyalgia.

Meal planning doesn't have to be complicated or time-consuming. Start small, with a few planned meals per week, and gradually build from there. To save you the time of planning your meal, there is an easy to follow meal plan included in this book.

Strategies for Batch Cooking and Prepping Meals in Advance

Batch cooking and meal prepping are lifesavers, allowing you to prepare delicious and healthy anti-inflammatory meals in advance. Here are some strategies to employ for a successful batch cooking and meal prepping:

Plan Your Meals

- **Choose a Dedicated Day:** Pick a day when you have good energy to cook and prepare meals for the week ahead.
- **Select Your Recipes:** Choose 2-3 recipes that are easy to prepare in bulk and freeze well.
- **Make a Shopping List:** List all the ingredients you'll need to minimize those energy-draining trips to the grocery store.

Batch Cooking

- **Double or Triple Recipes:** While you're cooking, double or triple your recipe to create extra portions for freezing. This saves time and ensures you have healthy meals readily available throughout the week.
- **Think Simmering Savory Delights:** Soups, stews, and chili are perfect for batch cooking. They freeze well and can be easily reheated for a satisfying meal.
- **Roast Up a Feast:** Roasting vegetables, chicken breasts, or salmon is another great option. Roasted veggies can be enjoyed hot or cold, and protein sources can be incorporated into various meals throughout the week.

How to Prep in Advance

- **Wash and Chop Veggies in Advance:** Wash and chop your vegetables on your high-energy day. Store them in airtight containers in the fridge for easy access throughout the week.
- **Pre-Cook Grains:** Cook a big pot of quinoa, brown rice, or lentils on your prep day. These pre-cooked grains can be used in various meals throughout the week.

- **Portion Control is Key:** Divide pre-cooked meals or ingredients into individual serving sizes and store them in airtight containers. This promotes portion control and makes grabbing a healthy meal even easier.

Freezing for Future Feasts

- **Invest in Freezer-Safe Containers:** Invest in a set of freezer-safe containers to store your prepped meals or cooked dishes.
- **Label Everything Clearly:** Don't forget to label your containers with the contents and date. This helps with organization and ensures you're rotating your frozen meals.
- **Reheating Tips:** When reheating frozen meals, thaw them in the refrigerator overnight for best results. You can also reheat them gently on the stovetop or microwave.

Bonus Tips

- **Cook Once, Eat Twice:** When cooking a protein source like chicken breasts, consider grilling or baking extras. You can use them in salads, sandwiches, or stir-fries throughout the week.
- **Delegate Tasks:** If you have a partner or family member who can help, delegate tasks like chopping vegetables or setting the table.
- **Listen to Your Body:** Prioritize rest. If you're feeling fatigued, don't push yourself. Batch cook or prep meals on a day when you have more energy.

By incorporating these batch cooking and meal prepping strategies, you're helping yourself to:

- Save time and energy in the kitchen.

- Reduce decision fatigue and stress about what to eat.

- Always have healthy and delicious options readily available.

- Manage your fibromyalgia symptoms by prioritizing a nutritious, anti-inflammatory diet.

Meal Plan Guide for Breakfast, Lunch, Dinner, Dessert and snacks tailored for fibromyalgia

This sample meal plan incorporates the anti-inflammatory recipes offered in this book with a variety for breakfast, lunch, dinner, desserts and snacks. Remember, this is just a sample, feel free to adjust portion sizes, ingredients, and recipes based on your preferences and dietary needs.

Week 1:

Breakfast:

- Day 1: Greek Yogurt with Berries and Chia Seeds

- Day 2: Edamame with Sea Salt

- Day 3: Roasted Sweet Potato with Nut Butter and Berries

- Day 4: Rice Cakes with Sliced Avocado and Smoked Salmon

- Day 5: Apple Slices with Almond Butter

- Day 6: Homemade Baked Applesauce

- Day 7: No-Bake Energy Bites with Dates and Nuts (prepare ahead for the week)

Lunch:

- Day 1: Bell Pepper Strips with Guacamole and a side salad

- Day 2: Sliced Vegetables with Cottage Cheese and whole-wheat crackers
- Day 3: Leftover Roasted Sweet Potato with a side salad
- Day 4: Trail Mix (pre-portion for grab-and-go lunches)
- Day 5: Cucumber Slices with Hummus and whole-wheat pita bread
- Day 6: Chickpea Salad Sandwich on whole-wheat bread (use leftover roasted chickpeas, chopped celery, red onion, light mayo, and seasonings)
- Day 7: Leftover soup or chili (opt for anti-inflammatory recipes)

Dinner:

- Day 1: Baked Salmon with Roasted Vegetables (use anti-inflammatory spices like turmeric and ginger)
- Day 2: Chicken Stir-fry with brown rice and mixed vegetables
- Day 3: Vegetarian Chili with whole-wheat bread
- Day 4: Lentil Soup with a side salad
- Day 5: Turkey Burgers on whole-wheat buns with sweet potato fries
- Day 6: Baked Tofu with roasted Brussels Sprouts and quinoa
- Day 7: Salmon with a side of roasted asparagus and quinoa

Dessert:

- Day 1: Roasted Chickpeas with Turmeric and Spices - This crunchy and protein-packed snack offers a satisfying sweet and savory flavor profile. The turmeric adds an anti-inflammatory boost.
- Day 2: Apple Slices with Almond Butter - A classic and simple option. Apples provide fiber and natural sweetness, while almond butter offers protein and healthy fats.

- Day 3: Greek Yogurt with Berries and Chia Seeds - This creamy and refreshing parfait is packed with protein, fiber, antioxidants, and healthy fats.
- Day 4: Bell Pepper Strips with Guacamole - While not traditionally considered a dessert, the sweetness of bell peppers combined with the creamy avocado in guacamole creates a unique and satisfying sweet and savory treat.
- Day 5: Trail Mix with Nuts, Seeds, and Dried Fruit - Customize your own mix with a variety of nuts, seeds, and dried fruits for a satisfying blend of protein, healthy fats, fiber, and natural sweetness.
- Day 6: Edamame with Sea Salt - This simple snack provides protein and fiber with a touch of salty sweetness.
- Day 7: Frozen Banana "Soft Serve" - Blend frozen bananas for a creamy, naturally sweet treat. You can add a drizzle of honey, nut butter, or chopped nuts for extra flavor and texture.

Snacks:

Throughout the week, enjoy any of the recipes mentioned above for snacks, like apple slices with almond butter, cucumber slices with hummus, or trail mix.

Week 2 & 3:

Follow a similar structure to Week 1, but swap out recipes for variety. Here are some ideas:

Breakfast:

- Oatmeal with berries and chopped nuts
- Scrambled eggs with spinach and whole-wheat toast
- Smoothie made with fruits, vegetables, and protein powder

Lunch:

- Tuna salad sandwich on whole-wheat bread with lettuce and tomato
- Leftover dinner from previous nights
- Lentil salad with chopped vegetables and a light vinaigrette Dinner
- Chicken breast with roasted sweet potato and steamed broccoli
- Shrimp scampi with whole-wheat pasta and a side salad
- Vegetarian lasagna made with lentil bolognese
- Black bean burgers on whole-wheat buns with a side salad

Dessert and Snacks:

Experiment with different fruits and vegetables throughout the week.

Week 4:

This week can focus on incorporating new recipes or revisiting favorites from the previous weeks. You can also use this week to plan meals around any dietary restrictions or preferences you may have.

Remember:

- This is a sample plan, adjust portion sizes and ingredients based on your needs.
- Drink plenty of water throughout the day.
- Consider incorporating anti-inflammatory beverages like green tea or turmeric tea.
- Consult a doctor or registered dietitian for personalized meal plan recommendations.
- Whenever possible, prepare meals in advance to save time during the week.
- Utilize leftovers for lunches or quick dinners.
- Get creative with spices and herbs to add flavor to your meals.
- Enjoy a variety of colorful fruits and vegetables throughout the week.
- Don't be afraid to experiment with new recipes.

Chapter 4: Deliciously Simple Recipes

Quick and Easy Breakfast Recipes

Berry Chia Pudding

A cool and refreshing breakfast parfait packed with protein, fiber, and antioxidants from berries and chia seeds.

Prep Time: 5 minutes

Cook Time: Overnight chilling

Servings: 1 serving (easily doubled)

Ingredients:

- ½ cup unsweetened nut milk (almond milk, cashew milk, etc.)
- ¼ cup chia seeds
- ¼ cup mixed berries (fresh or frozen)
- ¼ cup plain Greek yogurt (optional)
- Toppings (optional): Sliced almonds, chopped walnuts, a drizzle of honey

Instructions:

- In a small jar or container, whisk together the nut milk and chia seeds.
- Stir in the berries. If using frozen berries, let them thaw slightly before adding them.
- Cover the jar and refrigerate overnight or for at least 4 hours to allow the chia seeds to thicken.
- In the morning, top with yogurt (if using) and desired toppings.

Storage Tips: This chia pudding can be stored in the refrigerator for up to 3 days.

Nutritional Information: (Approximate per serving) Calories: 250, Protein: 5g, Fat: 10g, Carbohydrates: 25g (including fiber)

Scrambled Eggs with Spinach and Tomatoes

A protein-packed breakfast option with the added benefits of anti-inflammatory vegetables.

Prep Time: 5 minutes

Cook Time: 10 minutes

Servings: 1 serving (easily doubled)

Ingredients:

- 2 eggs
- 1 tablespoon olive oil
- ½ cup chopped spinach
- ¼ cup chopped tomato
- Salt and pepper to taste
- Optional additions: Chopped fresh herbs (parsley, chives), crumbled feta cheese

Instructions:

- Whisk together the eggs in a small bowl..
- Heat up olive oil in a pan over medium heat.
- Add the chopped spinach and cook until wilted, about 1 minute.
- Add the chopped tomatoes and cook for an additional minute.
- Pour the egg mixture into the pan and scramble the eggs to your desired consistency.
- Season with salt and pepper to taste.

- Serve immediately with optional additions.

Storage Tips: Leftovers can be stored in an airtight container in the refrigerator for up to 2 days. Reheat gently in a pan or microwave when using again.

Nutritional Information: (Approximate per serving): Calories: 250, Protein: 12g, Fat: 13g, Carbohydrates: 5g (including fiber)

Tropical Smoothie Bowl

A vibrant and delicious smoothie bowl packed with anti-inflammatory fruits and healthy fats.

Prep Time: 5 minutes

Cook Time: No cook

Servings: 1 serving (easily doubled)

Ingredients:

- ½ cup frozen mango chunks
- ½ cup frozen pineapple chunks
- ¼ cup unsweetened coconut milk
- ¼ cup plain Greek yogurt (optional)
- Toppings (optional): Sliced banana, chopped granola, a sprinkle of chia seeds

Instructions:

- Combine the frozen mango chunks, frozen pineapple chunks, coconut milk, and Greek yogurt (if using) in a blender
- Blend until smooth and creamy.
- Pour the smoothie into a bowl.
- Top with desired toppings.

Storage Tips: This smoothie bowl is best enjoyed fresh. Leftover smoothie can be stored in an airtight container in the freezer for up to 1 month. Thaw slightly before blending again and pouring into a bowl.

Nutritional Information: (Approximate per serving) Calories: 300, Protein: 5g (with Greek yogurt), Fat: 15g, Carbohydrates: 35g (including fiber)

Avocado Toast with Smoked Salmon

A simple and satisfying breakfast option with healthy fats from avocado and protein from smoked salmon.

Prep Time: 5 minutes

Cook Time: No cook

Servings: 1 serving (easily doubled)

Ingredients:

- 1 slice whole-wheat bread
- ½ ripe avocado, mashed
- 2 ounces smoked salmon
- Lemon juice (optional)
- Pinch of salt and pepper

Instructions:

- Toast the whole-wheat bread to your desired level of crispness.
- Spread the mashed avocado on the toast.
- Top with smoked salmon.
- Drizzle with a squeeze of lemon juice (optional) and season with a pinch of salt and pepper.

Storage Tips: This dish is best enjoyed fresh. Leftover avocado toast can be stored in an airtight container in the refrigerator for up to 1 day. However, the avocado may brown slightly.

Nutritional Information: (Approximate per serving) Calories: 350, Protein: 15g, Fat: 20g, Carbohydrates: 25g (including fiber)

Spiced Oatmeal with Berries and Nuts

A warm and comforting breakfast packed with fiber and anti-inflammatory benefits from berries and spices.

Prep Time: 5 minutes

Cook Time: 15 minutes

Servings: 1 serving (easily doubled)

Ingredients:

- ½ cup rolled oats
- 1 cup unsweetened nut milk (almond milk, cashew milk, etc.)
- ¼ cup water
- Pinch of ground cinnamon
- Pinch of ground ginger (optional)
- ¼ cup mixed berries (fresh or frozen)
- ¼ cup chopped nuts (almonds, walnuts, pecans)
- Maple syrup or honey (optional, to taste)

Instructions:

- In a small saucepan, combine oats, nut milk, water, cinnamon, and ginger (if using).
- Bring to a boil over medium heat.
- Reduce heat and simmer for 5-7 minutes, or until oats are cooked through and creamy, stirring occasionally.

- Remove from heat and stir in the berries. Let them sit for a minute to soften slightly.
- Top with chopped nuts and drizzle with maple syrup or honey (optional) to taste.

Storage Tips: Leftover oatmeal can be stored in an airtight container in the refrigerator for up to 3 days. Reheat gently using a saucepan or microwave when using again.

Nutritional Information: (Approximate per serving) Calories: 350, Protein: 5g, Fat: 15g, Carbohydrates: 40g (including fiber)

Greek Yogurt Parfait with Chia Seeds and Granola

A layered yogurt parfait with a satisfying combination of protein, fiber, and healthy fats.

Prep Time: 5 minutes

Cook Time: No cook

Servings: 1 serving (easily doubled)

Ingredients:

- ½ cup plain Greek yogurt
- ¼ cup chia seeds
- ¼ cup unsweetened nut milk (almond milk, cashew milk, etc.)
- ¼ cup granola
- ¼ cup fresh berries (optional)

Instructions:

- In a small glass or jar, layer half of the Greek yogurt.
- Sprinkle with half of the chia seeds.
- Pour in half of the nut milk.
- Add half of the granola.

- Repeat layers with remaining yogurt, chia seeds, nut milk, and granola.
- Top with fresh berries (optional).

Storage Tips: This parfait is best enjoyed fresh. Leftover parfait can be stored in an airtight container in the refrigerator for up to 2 days. The granola may become soft.

Nutritional Information: (Approximate per serving) Calories: 300, Protein: 15g, Fat: 10g, Carbohydrates: 30g (including fiber)

Salmon with Avocado Toast with Lime and Herbed Tahini Sauce

A flavorful and protein-packed breakfast with omega-3-rich salmon and a creamy avocado toast drizzle.

Prep Time: 5 minutes

Cook Time: 10 minutes

Servings: 1 serving (easily doubled)

Ingredients:

- 1 salmon fillet (about 4 oz)
- ½ avocado, mashed
- 2 tbsp chopped fresh parsley
- 1 tbsp fresh dill
- 1 tbsp lemon juice
- Salt and pepper to taste
- 1 tbsp olive oil
- 2 tbsp chopped fresh chives (optional)

Instructions:

- Preheat the oven to 400°F (200°C).
- Season salmon with salt and pepper.

- Drizzle with olive oil and spread with mashed avocado.
- Roast salmon for 10-12 minutes, or until cooked through and flakes easily.
- While salmon roasts, whip up a tahini sauce by combining tahini, olive oil, lemon juice, parsley, dill, salt, and pepper in a small bowl.
- Serve salmon on whole-wheat toast with a drizzle of the herb-tahini sauce.

Storage Tips: Store leftovers in an airtight plastic container placed in the refrigerator for up to three days.

Nutritional Information: (Approximate per serving) Calories: 350, Protein: 30g, Fat: 20g, Carbohydrates: 30g (including fiber)

Whole-Wheat Pancakes with Fruit and Coconut Yogurt

A simple and delicious breakfast option perfect for those who are gluten intolerant.

Prep Time: 15 minutes

Cook Time: 5 minutes

Servings: 2 servings

Ingredients:

- One and half cups of whole-wheat flour
- 1 cup buttermilk
- 2 large eggs
- 1/2 cup unsweetened coconut milk
- 1/2 tsp baking powder
- 1/4 tsp baking soda
- 1/4 tsp salt
- 1/4 cup fresh berries

- 1/4 cup coconut yogurt

Instructions:

- In a large bowl, whisk together flour, buttermilk, eggs, coconut milk, baking powder, baking soda, and salt.
- Add berries and coconut yogurt and mix until combined.
- Heat a griddle or pan over medium heat and cook pancakes for 2-3 minutes per side, or until golden brown.
- Serve pancakes with additional fruit and coconut yogurt, if desired.

Storage Tips: Leftover pancakes can be stored in an airtight container in the refrigerator for up to 3 days.

Nutritional Information: (Approximate per serving) Calories: 250, Protein: 20g, Fat: 15g, Carbohydrates: 30g (including fiber)

Tofu Scramble with Turmeric and Vegetables

A vegan twist on scrambled eggs, packed with protein and the anti-inflammatory benefits of turmeric.

Prep Time: 5 minutes

Cook Time: 10 minutes

Servings: 1 serving (easily doubled)

Ingredients:

- ¼ block firm tofu, crumbled
- ½ cup chopped vegetables (bell pepper, onion, mushrooms etc.)
- ¼ cup chopped spinach
- ¼ cup diced tomatoes
- 1 tbsp nutritional yeast
- ½ tsp turmeric powder
- Pinch of black pepper

- 1 tbsp olive oil

Instructions:

- Heat up olive oil in a pan over medium heat.
- Sauté chopped vegetables until softened, about 3-4 minutes.
- Add crumbled tofu and cook for an additional 2-3 minutes, allowing it to brown slightly.
- Stir in chopped spinach and diced tomatoes. Cook for another minute until spinach wilts.
- Sprinkle with nutritional yeast, turmeric powder, and black pepper. Toss to coat evenly.
- Serve immediately with whole-wheat toast or a side of greens.

Storage Tips: Store leftovers in an airtight plastic container in the refrigerator for up to two days. Reheat gently in a pan or microwave when using again.

Nutritional Information: (Approximate per serving) Calories: 300, Protein: 20g, Fat: 10g, Carbohydrates: 25g (including fiber)

Overnight Spiced Sweet Potato Oats

A delicious and nutritious breakfast option that can be prepared the night before for a grab-and-go meal.

Prep Time: 5 minutes

Cook Time: Overnight chilling

Servings: 1 serving (easily doubled)

Ingredients:

- ½ cup rolled oats
- ½ cup chopped sweet potato
- ½ cup unsweetened plant-based milk (almond milk, oat milk, etc.)

- ¼ cup chopped walnuts
- 1 tbsp chia seeds
- Pinch of ground cinnamon
- Pinch of ground ginger (optional)
- ¼ cup plain plant-based yogurt (optional)

Instructions:

- In a small jar or container, combine rolled oats, chopped sweet potato, plant-based milk, chopped walnuts, chia seeds, cinnamon, and ginger (if using).
- Stir well to combine and ensure all ingredients are coated.
- Cover the jar and refrigerate overnight for at least 4 hours, or up to overnight.
- In the morning, stir in plant-based yogurt (optional) and enjoy it chilled.

Storage Tips: This overnight oats recipe can be stored in the refrigerator for up to 3 days.

Nutritional Information: (Approximate per serving) Calories: 400, Protein: 5g (with yogurt), Fat: 20g, Carbohydrates: 50g (including fiber)

Quick and Easy Lunch Recipes

Mediterranean Tuna Salad with Whole-Wheat Pita

A protein-packed and flavorful lunch option with the added benefits of anti-inflammatory ingredients like olive oil and tomatoes.

Prep Time: 10 minutes

Cook Time: No cook

Servings: 1 serving (easily doubled)

Ingredients:

- 5 oz canned tuna (in water), drained
- ¼ cup chopped cucumber
- ¼ cup chopped tomato
- 1 tbsp chopped red onion
- 1 tbsp crumbled feta cheese (optional)
- 1 tbsp chopped fresh parsley
- 1 tbsp olive oil
- 1 tbsp lemon juice
- Salt and pepper to taste
- 1 whole-wheat pita bread

Instructions:

- Combine tuna, chopped cucumber, tomato, red onion, feta cheese (if using), and parsley in a bowl.
- Whisk together olive oil, lemon juice, salt, and pepper in a separate small bowl.
- Pour the dressing over the tuna salad mixture and toss to coat.
- Warm the whole-wheat pita bread according to package instructions (optional).
- Stuff the pita bread with the tuna salad mixture and enjoy.

Storage Tips: Leftover tuna salad can be stored in an airtight container in the refrigerator for up to 2 days. Store the pita bread separately.

Nutritional Information: (Approximate per serving) Calories: 400, Protein: 30g, Fat: 15g, Carbohydrates: 30g (including fiber)

Lentil Soup with Greens and Lemon

A hearty and satisfying soup packed with protein and fiber from lentils,
perfect for a light and anti-inflammatory lunch.

Prep Time: 10 minutes

Cook Time: 20 minutes

Servings: 1 serving (easily doubled)

Ingredients:

- ½ cup brown lentils, rinsed
- 1 cup vegetable broth
- ½ cup chopped spinach
- ¼ cup chopped carrots
- 1 clove garlic, minced
- 1 tbsp olive oil
- Juice of ½ lemon
- Salt and pepper to taste

Instructions:

- Heat up olive oil in a saucepan over medium heat.
- Add chopped garlic and cook for up to 30 seconds, until fragrant.
- Add chopped carrots and saute for another minute.
- Stir in rinsed lentils and vegetable broth.
- Bring to a boiling point, then reduce heat and simmer for 15 to 20 minutes, or until lentils are tender.
- Stir in chopped spinach and lemon juice. Cook for an additional minute, until spinach wilts.
- Season with salt and pepper to taste.

Storage Tips: Store leftover soup in an airtight plastic container in the refrigerator for up to three days.

Nutritional Information: (Approximate per serving) Calories: 250, Protein: 15g, Fat: 5g, Carbohydrates: 35g (including fiber)

Chicken and Veggie Buddha Bowl with Turmeric Tahini Sauce

A vibrant and customizable lunch bowl packed with protein, vegetables, and a creamy turmeric-infused tahini sauce.

Prep Time: 15 minutes

Cook Time: 10 minutes (depending on chosen protein)

Servings: 1 serving (easily doubled)

Ingredients:

- 4 oz cooked chicken breast (grilled, baked, or poached)
- ½ cup chopped vegetables (broccoli, cauliflower, bell peppers, etc.)
- ¼ cup cooked brown rice or quinoa
- ¼ cup chopped baby spinach or arugula
- 2 tbsp crumbled feta cheese (optional)
- Chopped fresh herbs (parsley, cilantro, optional)

For the Turmeric Tahini Sauce:

- 2 tbsp tahini
- 1 tbsp olive oil
- 1 tbsp lemon juice
- ¼ cup water
- ½ tsp ground turmeric
- Pinch of salt and pepper

Instructions:

- Prepare the sauce: In a small bowl, whisk together tahini, olive oil, lemon juice, water, turmeric, salt, and pepper until smooth and creamy.
- Cook protein (if not already cooked): If using raw chicken breast, grill, bake, or poach it until cooked through. Shred or slice the cooked chicken.
- Assemble the bowl: Divide cooked brown rice or quinoa, chopped vegetables, and baby spinach or arugula between bowls.
- Top with sliced or shredded chicken and crumbled feta cheese (if using).
- Drizzle with desired amount of turmeric tahini sauce.
- Garnish with chopped fresh herbs (optional).

Storage Tips: Leftover cooked chicken and sauce can be stored in separate airtight containers in the refrigerator for up to 3 days. Store other bowl components separately and assemble fresh when ready to eat.

Nutritional Information: (Approximate per serving, without feta cheese) Calories: 400, Protein: 30g, Fat: 15g, Carbohydrates: 35g (including fiber)

Salmon Salad Sandwich with Avocado and Whole-Wheat Bread

A delicious and satisfying sandwich option with omega-3-rich salmon and the healthy fats of avocado.

Prep Time: 10 minutes

Cook Time: No cook (if using pre-cooked salmon)

Servings: 1 serving (easily doubled)

Ingredients:

- 2 slices whole-wheat bread

- 3 oz cooked salmon (grilled, baked, or poached)
- ½ avocado, mashed
- 1 tbsp chopped red onion (optional)
- 1 tbsp fresh dill (optional)
- Squeeze of lemon juice
- Salt and pepper to taste

Instructions:

- Toast the whole-wheat bread to your desired level of crispness.
- Spread mashed avocado on both slices of toast.
- Flake cooked salmon and arrange it on one slice of toast.
- Top with chopped red onion (optional) and fresh dill (optional).
- Drizzle with a squeeze of lemon juice and season with salt and pepper to taste.
- Top with the other slice of avocado toast and enjoy.

Storage Tips: Leftover sandwiches can be wrapped tightly in plastic wrap or stored in an airtight container in the refrigerator for up to 1 day. The avocado may brown slightly.

Nutritional Information: (Approximate per serving) Calories: 450, Protein: 30g, Fat: 20g, Carbohydrates: 40g (including fiber)

Lentil and Veggie Wrap with Tzatziki Sauce

A protein-packed and portable lunch option featuring lentils, colorful veggies, and a refreshing homemade tzatziki sauce.

Prep Time: 15 minutes

Cook Time: 20 minutes (depending on chosen cooking method for lentils)

Servings: 1 serving (easily doubled)

Ingredients:

- ½ cup cooked green lentils
- ½ cup chopped vegetables (cucumber, bell peppers, carrots, etc.)
- ¼ cup chopped romaine lettuce
- 2 tbsp crumbled feta cheese (optional)
- 1 whole wheat tortilla

For the Tzatziki Sauce:

- ½ cup plain Greek yogurt
- 1 small cucumber, grated
- 1 tbsp olive oil
- 1 tbsp chopped fresh dill
- 1 clove garlic, minced
- Pinch of salt and pepper

Instructions:

- Prepare the tzatziki sauce: Combine Greek yogurt, grated cucumber, olive oil, chopped dill, minced garlic, salt, and pepper in a small bowl. Stir well and refrigerate for at least 15 minutes to allow flavors to meld.
- Cook lentils (if not already cooked): If using dry lentils, rinse and cook them according to package instructions until tender.
- Assemble the wrap: Spread a layer of tzatziki sauce on a whole wheat tortilla.
- Top with chopped romaine lettuce, cooked lentils, and chopped vegetables.
- Sprinkle with crumbled feta cheese (optional).
- Fold the bottom of the tortilla up and over the filling, then roll tightly to close.

Storage Tips: Store leftover cooked lentils and tzatziki sauce in separate airtight containers in the refrigerator for up to three days. Store the wrap separately and assemble fresh when ready to eat.

Nutritional Information: (Approximate per serving, without feta cheese) Calories: 350, Protein: 15g, Fat: 10g, Carbohydrates: 40g (including fiber)

Quinoa Salad with Roasted Vegetables and Lemon Vinaigrette

A light and flavorful salad packed with protein from quinoa, roasted vegetables, and a tangy lemon vinaigrette.

Prep Time: 15 minutes

Cook Time: 20 minutes for roasting vegetables + 15 minutes for cooking quinoa

Servings: 1 serving (easily doubled)

Ingredients:

- ½ cup cooked quinoa
- ½ cup roasted vegetables (broccoli, cauliflower, sweet potato, etc.)
- ¼ cup chopped cucumber
- ¼ cup crumbled feta cheese (optional)
- Chopped fresh herbs (parsley, mint, optional)

For the Lemon Vinaigrette:

- 1 tbsp olive oil
- 1 tbsp lemon juice
- 1 tsp honey
- Pinch of salt and pepper

Instructions:

- Roast vegetables: Preheat the oven to 400°F (200°C). Prepare your chosen vegetables by chopping them into bite-sized pieces. Drizzle with olive oil, salt, and pepper and toss gently. Roast on a baking sheet for 15-20 minutes, or until tender and slightly browned.
- Cook quinoa (if not already cooked): Rinse quinoa and cook it according to package instructions until fluffy.
- Prepare the vinaigrette: In a small bowl, whisk together olive oil, lemon juice, honey, salt, and pepper.
- Assemble the salad: In a bowl, combine cooked quinoa, roasted vegetables, chopped cucumber, and crumbled feta cheese (optional).
- Drizzle with desired amount of lemon vinaigrette and toss to coat.
- Garnish with chopped fresh herbs (optional).

Storage Tips: Leftover cooked quinoa, roasted vegetables, and vinaigrette can be stored in separate airtight containers in the refrigerator for up to 3 days. Store other salad components separately and assemble fresh when ready to eat.

Nutritional Information: (Approximate per serving, without feta cheese) Calories: 400, Protein: 10g, Fat: 15g, Carbohydrates: 50g (including fiber)

Black Bean Burgers with Spicy Salsa

These flavorful and protein-packed patties are packed with fiber and taste surprisingly delicious with the added kick of jalapenos. The spicy salsa adds a nice spicy contrast to the savory black bean flavor.

Prep Time: 10 minutes

Cook Time: 15 minutes (oven-baked)

Servings: 1 serving (easily doubled)

Ingredients:

- 1 can black beans, drained and rinsed
- 1/2 cup cooked quinoa or brown rice
- 1/4 cup chopped onion
- 1/4 cup chopped jalapenos (adjust jalapeno according to spice preference)
- 1/4 cup mashed avocado
- 1/2 cup breadcrumbs
- 1 egg
- 1 tbsp olive oil
- Salt and pepper to taste

For the Spicy Salsa:

- 2 tomatoes, finely chopped
- 1/2 red onion, finely chopped
- 1 serrano pepper, seeded and finely chopped (adjust according to spice preference)
- 1/2 cup cilantro, chopped
- 1/2 avocado, diced
- 1 tbsp lime juice
- 1 tbsp olive oil
- Salt and pepper to taste

Instructions:

- Combine all black bean ingredients in a large bowl and mix well.
- Divide into 4 patties and season with salt and pepper to taste.
- Preheat the oven to 400°F (200°C).

- Place patties on a baking sheet lined with parchment paper and bake for 15 minutes per side, or until cooked through and browned.
- Prepare the salsa: In a small bowl, combine all salsa ingredients and mix well.
- Serve black bean burgers with the spicy salsa.

Storage Tips: Store leftover black bean burgers and salsa in an airtight container in the refrigerator for up to three days.

Nutritional Information: (Approximate per serving) Calories: 450, Protein: 25g, Fat: 15g, Carbohydrates: 35g (including fiber)

Salmon Foil Boats with Avocado Salsa

These easy and healthy salmon dishes are packed with protein and are perfect for a quick weeknight meal. The avocado salsa adds a creamy and delicious counterpoint to the rich salmon flavor.

Prep Time: 15 minutes

Cook Time: 15 minutes (per salmon)

Servings: 1 serving (easily doubled)

Ingredients:

- 2 salmon fillets (about 4 oz each)
- 4 sheets parchment paper
- 2 tbsp avocado, mashed
- 1 tbsp olive oil
- Salt and pepper to taste

For the Avocado Salsa:

- 1 red onion, finely chopped
- 1 serrano pepper, seeded and finely chopped (adjust according to spice preference)

- 2 jalapenos, seeded and finely chopped (adjust according to spice preference)
- 1 clove garlic, minced
- 1/2 cup cilantro, chopped
- 1/4 cup red onion, chopped (optional)
- 1/4 cup lime juice
- 1 tbsp olive oil
- Salt and pepper to taste

Instructions:

- Preheat the oven to 400°F (200°C).
- Place each salmon fillet on a sheet of parchment paper, skin side down.
- Spread mashed avocado on the salmon fillet. Season with salt and pepper.
- Place the salmon fillet on the other side of the parchment paper, creating a boat shape.
- Drizzle with olive oil.
- Fold the parchment paper around the salmon filet to create a tight boat.
- Bake for 15 minutes per salmon, or until cooked through and browned.
- While the salmon cooks, prepare the avocado salsa.
- To make the salsa, combine all salsa ingredients and mix well.
- To serve, remove salmon from the oven and carefully open the boat to expose the salmon. Drizzle with avocado salsa and serve immediately.

Storage Tips: Store leftover salmon dishes in an airtight container in the refrigerator for up to three days. The avocado salsa can also be made ahead of time and stored in the refrigerator for up to five. days.

Nutritional Information: (Approximate per serving) Calories: 400, Protein: 30g, Fat: 20g, Carbohydrates: 35g (including fiber)

Turkey and Veggie Meatballs with Marinara Sauce

A healthier twist on classic meatballs, featuring lean ground turkey and a medley of colorful vegetables. Served with a simple marinara sauce for a satisfying and protein-packed lunch.

Prep Time: 15 minutes

Cook Time: 20 minutes (baking) + 10 minutes (simmering sauce - optional)

Servings: 1 serving (easily doubled)

Ingredients:

- ½ pound lean ground turkey
- ½ cup chopped vegetables (bell peppers, mushrooms, zucchini, etc.)
- ¼ cup panko breadcrumbs
- 1 tbsp grated Parmesan cheese
- 1 tbsp chopped fresh parsley
- 1 egg
- 1 tsp dried oregano
- ½ tsp garlic powder
- Salt and pepper to taste

For the Marinara Sauce (Optional):

- 1 can (14.5 oz) crushed tomatoes
- 1 tbsp olive oil

- 1 tsp dried oregano
- Pinch of red pepper flakes (optional)
- Salt and pepper to taste

Instructions:

- Preheat the oven to 400°F (200°C).
- Combine ground turkey, chopped vegetables, panko breadcrumbs, Parmesan cheese, parsley, egg, oregano, garlic powder, salt, and pepper in a large bowl. Mix well until combined.
- Shape the mixture into small meatballs.
- Arrange meatballs on a baking sheet covered with parchment paper.
- Bake for about 20 minutes, or until cooked through and brown in color.

For the Marinara Sauce (Optional):

- While the meatballs bake, heat olive oil in a saucepan over medium heat.
- Add crushed tomatoes, oregano, and red pepper flakes (if using).
- Cook for 10 minutes, stirring occasionally. Season with salt and pepper to taste.

Assembly:

- Serve baked meatballs on a plate with your desired amount of marinara sauce (optional).

Storage Tips: Store leftover meatballs and marinara sauce in separate airtight containers in the refrigerator for up to three days.

Nutritional Information: (Approximate per serving, without marinara sauce) Calories: 400, Protein: 30g, Fat: 15g, Carbohydrates: 25g (including fiber)

Chicken Caesar Salad with a Twist

A lighter take on the classic Caesar salad, featuring grilled chicken, romaine lettuce, and a creamy avocado-based dressing.

Prep Time: 10 minutes

Cook Time: No cook (if using pre-cooked chicken)

Servings: 1 serving (easily doubled)

Ingredients:

- 2 cups chopped romaine lettuce
- 3 oz cooked chicken breast (grilled, baked, or poached)
- ¼ cup cherry tomatoes, halved
- ¼ cup grated Parmesan cheese
- 2 tbsp crumbled whole-wheat crackers

For the Avocado Caesar Dressing:

- 1/2 ripe avocado, mashed
- 1 tbsp olive oil
- 1 tbsp lemon juice
- 1 tbsp water
- 1 tsp Dijon mustard
- 1/4 tsp garlic powder
- Pinch of salt and pepper

Instructions:

- ***Prepare the dressing:*** In a blender or food processor, combine mashed avocado, olive oil, lemon juice, water, Dijon mustard, garlic powder, salt, and pepper. Blend until smooth and creamy.
- ***Assemble the salad:*** In a large bowl, toss together romaine lettuce, chopped chicken breast, cherry tomatoes, and Parmesan cheese.

- Drizzle with desired amount of avocado Caesar dressing and toss to coat.
- Top with crumbled whole-wheat crackers for a crunchy texture.

Storage Tips: Store leftover cooked chicken and dressing in separate airtight containers in the refrigerator for up to three days. Store other salad components separately and assemble fresh when ready to eat.

Nutritional Information: (Approximate per serving) Calories: 400, Protein: 30g, Fat: 20g, Carbohydrates: 20g (including fiber)

Quick and Easy Dinner Recipes

Sheet Pan Salmon with Roasted Vegetables and Lemon Herb Drizzle

A fuss-free and flavorful dinner featuring omega-3-rich salmon baked alongside colorful vegetables. The lemon herb drizzle adds a bright and zesty touch.

Prep Time: 15 minutes

Cook Time: 20-25 minutes

Servings: 1 serving (easily doubled)

Ingredients:

- 4 oz salmon fillet
- ½ cup chopped vegetables (broccoli, cauliflower, zucchini, etc.)
- 1 tbsp olive oil
- Salt and pepper to taste

For the Lemon Herb Drizzle:

- 1 tbsp olive oil
- 1 tbsp lemon juice

- 1 tsp chopped fresh parsley
- 1 tsp chopped fresh dill
- Pinch of garlic powder

Instructions:

- Preheat the oven to 400°F (200°C).
- Combine chopped vegetables with olive oil, salt, and pepper. Spread the mixture out on a baking sheet.
- Place salmon fillet on top of the vegetables.
- In a small bowl, whisk together olive oil, lemon juice, parsley, dill, and garlic powder to create the lemon herb drizzle.
- Drizzle the lemon herb drizzle over the salmon.
- Bake for 20-25 minutes, or until salmon is cooked through and vegetables are tender-crisp.

Storage Tips: Store leftover salmon and vegetables in an airtight container in the refrigerator for up to three days.

Nutritional Information: (Approximate per serving) Calories: 450, Protein: 30g, Fat: 25g, Carbohydrates: 20g (including fiber)

One-Pot Chicken and Veggie Quinoa Bowl with Turmeric Coconut Curry

A hearty and satisfying bowl packed with protein, vegetables, and a fragrant turmeric coconut curry. Made in one pot for easy clean-up.

Prep Time: 10 minutes

Cook Time: 25 minutes

Servings: 1 serving (easily doubled)

Ingredients:

- 4 oz boneless, skinless chicken breast (cubed)

- ½ cup chopped vegetables (broccoli, carrots, bell peppers, etc.)
- ¼ cup quinoa, rinsed
- 1 cup coconut milk
- ½ cup vegetable broth
- 1 tbsp curry powder
- ½ tsp ground turmeric
- Salt and pepper to taste

Instructions:

- In a large pot or Dutch oven, heat a bit of oil over medium heat. Add cubed chicken and cook until browned on all sides.
- Stir in chopped vegetables and cook for an additional 2-3 minutes, or until slightly softened.
- Add rinsed quinoa, coconut milk, vegetable broth, curry powder, turmeric, salt, and pepper.
- Bring to a boil, then reduce heat and simmer for 15-20 minutes, or until quinoa is cooked through and liquid is absorbed.
- To achieve desired taste, season with additional salt and pepper.

Storage Tips: Store leftover chicken and quinoa mixture in an airtight container in the refrigerator for up to three days.

Nutritional Information: (Approximate per serving) Calories: 400, Protein: 30g, Fat: 15g, Carbohydrates: 35g (including fiber)

Shrimp Scampi with Zucchini Noodles

A lighter take on a classic dish, featuring succulent shrimp tossed in a flavorful garlic butter sauce with zucchini noodles for a satisfying and low-carb option.

Prep Time: 10 minutes

Cook Time: 10 minutes

Servings: 1 serving (easily doubled)

Ingredients:

- 5 oz peeled and deveined shrimp
- 1 tbsp olive oil
- 2 cloves garlic, minced
- 1 tbsp chopped fresh parsley
- 1/4 cup dry white wine (optional)
- 1/4 cup chicken broth
- 1 tbsp lemon juice
- 1/2 tsp red pepper flakes (optional)
- Salt and pepper to taste
- 1 medium zucchini, spiralized (or use store-bought zucchini noodles)

Instructions:

- In a large skillet, heat up olive oil over medium heat. Add shrimp and cook each side for 2-3 minutes, or until pink and opaque. Remove the shrimp from the pan and keep it aside.
- Add chopped garlic to the pan and cook for 30 seconds, until fragrant. Be careful not to burn the garlic.
- Stir in chopped parsley, white wine (if using), chicken broth, lemon juice, and red pepper flakes (if using). Cook for 2 to 3 minutes, or until a little bit reduced.
- Use salt and pepper for seasoning to achieve the desired taste.
- Add cooked shrimp back to the pan and toss gently to coat in the sauce.
- While the sauce simmers, spiralize the zucchini or use store-bought zucchini noodles.

- Heat a separate pan over medium heat and cook the zucchini noodles for 1-2 minutes, or until slightly softened.
- Serve shrimp scampi over zucchini noodles and spoon the sauce over the top.

Storage Tips: Store leftover shrimp and sauce in an airtight container in the refrigerator for up to one day. Zucchini noodles are best served fresh, but leftover cooked zucchini noodles can be stored in the refrigerator for up to 2 days.

Nutritional Information: (Approximate per serving) Calories: 350, Protein: 30g, Fat: 15g, Carbohydrates: 15g (including fiber)

Turkey Meatloaf with Sweet Potato Mash

A comforting and healthy take on meatloaf, featuring lean ground turkey and topped with a delicious and nutritious sweet potato mash.

Prep Time: 15 minutes

Cook Time: 40 minutes

Servings: 1 serving (easily doubled)

Ingredients:

- ½ pound lean ground turkey
- ¼ cup chopped onion
- ¼ cup chopped mushrooms
- ¼ cup chopped bell pepper
- ¼ cup panko breadcrumbs
- 1 tbsp chopped fresh parsley
- 1 tbsp Worcestershire sauce
- 1 egg
- Salt and pepper to taste

-
- For the Sweet Potato Mash:
- 1 medium sweet potato, peeled and diced
- 1/4 cup water
- 1 tbsp olive oil
- Salt and pepper to taste

Instructions:

- Preheat the oven to 375°F (190°C).
- Combine ground turkey, chopped onion, mushrooms, bell pepper, panko breadcrumbs, parsley, Worcestershire sauce, egg, salt, and pepper in a large bowl. Mix thoroughly until combined.
- Shape the mixture into a loaf and place on a baking sheet.
- Bake for 30 minutes.

For the Sweet Potato Mash:

- While the meatloaf bakes, transfer the diced sweet potato and water in a saucepan. Bring to a boil, then reduce heat and simmer for 10 to 15 minutes, or until sweet potatoes are tender.
- Drain the excess water from the potatoes
- Mash the sweet potatoes with olive oil, salt, and pepper.

Assembly:

- After 30 minutes, remove the meatloaf from the oven and top with the sweet potato mash.
- Take it back to the oven and bake for an additional 10 minutes, or until the meatloaf is thoroughly cooked.

Storage Tips: Store leftover meatloaf and sweet potato mash in separate airtight containers in the refrigerator for up to three days.

Nutritional Information: (Approximate per serving) Calories: 450, Protein: 35g, Fat: 20g, Carbohydrates: 30g (including fiber)

Lentil Shepherd's Pie with Cauliflower Mash

A hearty and satisfying vegetarian twist on the classic shepherd's pie. Lentils replace ground lamb, offering a protein-rich alternative, while creamy cauliflower mash takes the place of traditional mashed potatoes.

Prep Time: 15 minutes

Cook Time: 30 minutes

Servings: 1 serving (easily doubled)

Ingredients:

- ½ cup brown lentils, rinsed
- 1 cup vegetable broth
- ½ cup chopped vegetables (carrots, peas, celery, etc.)
- 1 tbsp olive oil
- 1 tbsp tomato paste
- ½ tsp dried thyme
- Salt and pepper to taste

For the Cauliflower Mash:

- 1 cup cauliflower florets, chopped
- ¼ cup unsweetened almond milk (or milk of choice)
- 1 tbsp butter
- Salt and pepper to taste

Instructions:

- ***Prepare the lentils:*** Combine brown lentils, vegetable broth, and a pinch of salt In a saucepan. Bring to a boiling point, then reduce heat and simmer for 20-25 minutes, or until lentils are tender.

- While the lentils cook, heat up olive oil in a skillet over medium heat. Add chopped vegetables and cook for 5-7 minutes, or until softened.
- Stir in tomato paste, dried thyme, and salt and pepper to taste. Cook for an additional minute.
- Once lentils are cooked, drain any excess water and add them to the skillet with the vegetables. Stir thoroughly to combine.

For the Cauliflower Mash:

- Steam or boil cauliflower florets until tender, about 10 minutes.
- Drain any excess water from the cauliflower.
- Melt butter over medium heat in a small saucepan. Add mashed cauliflower, almond milk (or milk of choice), salt, and pepper to taste. Mash until smooth and creamy.

Assembly:

- Preheat the oven to 375°F (190°C).
- Transfer the lentil mixture to an oven-safe dish. Top with the cauliflower mash.
- Bake for 10-15 minutes, or until heated through and the top is slightly golden brown.

Storage Tips: Store leftover lentil mixture and cauliflower mash in separate airtight containers in the refrigerator for up to three days.

Nutritional Information: (Approximate per serving) Calories: 400, Protein: 15g, Fat: 15g, Carbohydrates: 40g (including fiber)

Salmon with Roasted Brussels Sprouts and Lemon Dill Sauce

A simple and flavorful dish featuring omega-3-rich salmon roasted alongside Brussels sprouts and drizzled with a refreshing lemon dill sauce.

Prep Time: 10 minutes

Cook Time: 20 minutes

Servings: 1 serving (easily doubled)

Ingredients:

- 4 oz salmon fillet
- ½ cup Brussels sprouts, trimmed and halved
- 1 tbsp olive oil
- Salt and pepper to taste

For the Lemon Dill Sauce:

- 1 tbsp olive oil
- 1 tbsp lemon juice
- 1 tsp chopped fresh dill
- Pinch of garlic powder
- Salt and pepper to taste

Instructions:

- Preheat the oven to 400°F (200°C).
- Gently toss Brussels sprouts with olive oil, salt, and pepper. Arrange a baking sheet and spread the mixture out on it.
- Place salmon fillet on a separate baking sheet.
- Bake both the Brussels sprouts and salmon for 15-20 minutes, or until salmon is cooked through and Brussels sprouts are tender-crisp.

For the Lemon Dill Sauce:

- While the salmon and Brussels sprouts cook, whisk together olive oil, lemon juice, chopped dill, garlic powder, salt, and pepper in a small bowl.

Assembly:

- Once cooked, plate the salmon and roasted Brussels sprouts.
- Drizzle the lemon dill sauce over the salmon and enjoy.

Storage Tips: Store leftover salmon and roasted Brussels sprouts in an airtight container in the refrigerator for up to three days. The lemon dill sauce is best served fresh.

Nutritional Information: (Approximate per serving) Calories: 400, Protein: 30g, Fat: 20g, Carbohydrates: 20g (including fiber)

One-Pan Chicken and Veggie Quinoa Bowl with Turmeric Coconut Curry

This quick and easy one-pan chicken and veggie quinoa bowl is perfect for busy weeknights. The turmeric coconut curry adds a delicious and comforting flavor that's perfect for a plant-based meal.

Prep Time: 10 minutes

Cook Time: 25 minutes

Servings: 1 serving (easily doubled)

Ingredients:

- 4 oz boneless, skinless chicken breast (cubed)
- ½ cup chopped vegetables (broccoli, carrots, bell peppers, etc.)
- ¼ cup quinoa, rinsed
- 1 cup coconut milk
- ½ cup vegetable broth
- 1 tbsp curry powder
- ½ tsp ground turmeric
- Salt and pepper to taste
- 1 medium zucchini, spiralized (or use store-bought zucchini noodles)

Instructions:

- In a large pot or Dutch oven, heat a bit of oil over medium heat. Add cubed chicken and cook until browned on all sides.

- Stir in chopped vegetables (broccoli, carrots, bell peppers, etc.) and cook for an additional 2-3 minutes, or until slightly softened.
- Add rinsed quinoa to the pot along with coconut milk, vegetable broth, curry powder, turmeric, salt, and pepper.
- Bring to a boil, then reduce heat and simmer for 15-20 minutes, or until quinoa is cooked through and liquid is absorbed.
- Season with additional salt and pepper to achieve desired taste (optional).

Storage Tips: Store leftover shrimp and sauce in an airtight container in the refrigerator for up to 1 day. Zucchini noodles are best served fresh, but leftover cooked zucchini noodles can be stored in the refrigerator for up to 2 days.

Nutritional Information: (Approximate per serving) Calories: 350, Protein: 30g, Fat: 15g, Carbohydrates: 15g (including fiber)

Roasted Chicken Thighs with Sweet Potatoes and Broccolini

This dish is a healthy and satisfying option for a meal with family. The chicken thighs are roasted in a flavorful mixture of olive oil, spices, and herbs, while the sweet potatoes and broccoli are roasted to perfection.

Prep Time: 20 minutes

Cook Time: 30 minutes

Servings: 4 servings (easily doubled)

Ingredients:

- 4 bone-in, skin-on chicken thighs, about 1 pound each
- 1 tablespoon olive oil
- 1 teaspoon garlic powder
- 1/2 teaspoon salt

- 1/4 teaspoon black pepper
- 1 peeled medium sweet potato cut into chunks
- 1 bunch broccoli florets, trimmed
- 1 cup unsweetened almond milk (or milk of choice)

Instructions:

- Preheat the oven to 400°F (200°C).
- Whisk together olive oil, garlic powder, salt, and pepper in a small bowl. Brush the mixture generously over chicken thighs.
- Arrange chicken thighs in a single layer on a baking sheet.
- Place sweet potato chunks and broccoli florets on top of the chicken thighs.
- Drizzle the remaining olive oil mixture over the chicken and vegetables.
- Bake for 20 minutes, or until chicken is cooked through and vegetables are tender-crisp.
- Add almond milk (or milk of choice) to the baking sheet and stir to coat the chicken and vegetables.
- Bake for an additional 10-15 minutes, or until almond milk has evaporated and the vegetables are very tender.

Storage Tips: Store leftover chicken thighs and sweet potato and broccoli mixture in separate airtight containers in the refrigerator for up to 3 days.

Nutritional Information: (Approximate per serving) Calories: 550, Protein: 40g, Fat: 30g, Carbohydrates: 40g (including fiber)

- **Please note:** This is an estimate and the actual nutritional information may vary depending on the size of the chicken thighs, the amount of olive oil used, and the specific type of milk used.

Curried Lentil Soup with Coconut Milk and Greens

This hearty and flavorful soup is packed with protein and fiber from lentils, and the creamy coconut milk adds a touch of sweetness. Plus, it's easily doubled for those living with fibromyalgia who might want leftovers for another meal.

Prep Time: 15 minutes

Cook Time: 30 minutes

Servings: 1 serving (easily doubled)

Ingredients:

- ½ cup brown lentils, rinsed
- 1 cup vegetable broth
- ½ cup chopped vegetables (carrots, celery, onion, etc.)
- 1 tbsp olive oil
- 1 tsp curry powder
- ½ tsp ground turmeric
- 1 (13.5 oz) can coconut milk (light or full-fat)
- 2 cups chopped kale or spinach
- Salt and pepper to taste

Instructions:

- Heat up olive oil over medium heat in a pot or large saucepan. Add chopped vegetables and cook for 5-7 minutes, or until softened.
- Stir in rinsed lentils, curry powder, and turmeric. Cook for an additional minute, allowing the spices to toast.
- Pour in vegetable broth and coconut milk. Bring to a boiling point, then reduce heat and simmer for 20-25 minutes, or until lentils are tender.

- Add chopped kale or spinach and cook for an additional 2-3 minutes, or until wilted.
- Use salt and pepper as seasoning to achieve the desired taste.

Storage Tips: Store leftover soup in an airtight container in the refrigerator for up to three days.

Nutritional Information: (Approximate per serving) Calories: 350, Protein: 15g, Fat: 15g, Carbohydrates: 35g (including fiber)

Salmon with Lemon-Herb Butter and Roasted Asparagus

This simple and elegant dish features omega-3-rich salmon baked with a flavorful lemon-herb butter and paired with roasted asparagus. It's a quick and delicious meal perfect for a busy week's dinner.

Prep Time: 10 minutes

Cook Time: 20 minutes

Servings: 1 serving (easily doubled)

Ingredients:

- 4 oz salmon fillet
- 1 tbsp butter, softened
- 1 tbsp chopped fresh parsley
- 1 tsp lemon juice
- Pinch of garlic powder
- ½ bunch asparagus, trimmed
- Salt and pepper to taste

Instructions:

- Preheat the oven to 400°F (200°C).
- Mash together softened butter, chopped parsley, lemon juice, and garlic powder in a small bowl to create a lemon-herb butter.

- Arrange salmon fillet on a baking sheet lined with parchment paper. Season with salt and pepper.
- Top the salmon with the lemon-herb butter.
- Gently toss asparagus with a bit of olive oil, salt, and pepper. Spread the tossed mixture out on a separate baking sheet.
- Bake the salmon for 15-20 minutes, or until cooked thoroughly. Bake the asparagus for the last 10 minutes of cooking time for the salmon.

Storage Tips: Store leftover salmon and roasted asparagus in separate airtight containers in the refrigerator for up to three days.

Nutritional Information: (Approximate per serving) Calories: 400, Protein: 30g, Fat: 25g, Carbohydrates: 15g (including fiber)

Anti-Inflammatory Desserts Recipes

Dark Chocolate Avocado Mousse

This decadent mousse is a healthy and delicious alternative to traditional desserts. Creamy avocados and rich dark chocolate combine to create a satisfying treat that's also good for you. Plus, it's packed with healthy fats and antioxidants, making it a great choice for individuals with fibromyalgia.

Prep Time: 10 minutes

Servings: 2 (easily doubled)

Ingredients:

- 1 ripe avocado, halved and pitted
- 4 oz dark chocolate (at least 70% cacao), melted
- 1/4 cup unsweetened almond milk or any milk of choice.
- 1 tbsp maple syrup (or honey)

- 1/2 tsp vanilla extract
- Pinch of sea salt

Instructions:

- In a blender or food processor, combine the avocado flesh, melted dark chocolate, almond milk, maple syrup, vanilla extract, and salt. Blend until the texture turns smooth and creamy, scrape down the sides of the blender as needed.
- Taste and adjust sweetness as desired.
- Divide the mousse between two serving glasses or bowls.
- Place in the refrigerator for at least 30 minutes to chill before serving.

Storage Tips: Store leftover mousse in an airtight container in the refrigerator for up to two days. However, the avocado may start to turn brown.

Nutritional Information: (Approximate per serving) Calories: 350, Protein: 4g, Fat: 25g (including healthy fats from avocado), Carbohydrates: 20g (including fiber)

Additional Tips:

- For a richer flavor, use dark chocolate with a higher cacao content.
- You can top the mousse with a variety of things, such as fresh berries, chopped nuts, shredded coconut, or a sprinkle of cocoa powder.
- If you don't have a blender or food processor, you can mash the avocado with a fork and then whisk it together with the melted chocolate and other ingredients. However, the texture may not be as smooth.

Chia Seed Pudding with Berries and Nuts

This chia seed pudding is a fiber-rich and satisfying dessert that's perfect for meal prepping. Packed with antioxidants from berries and healthy fats from nuts, it's a delicious and anti-inflammatory treat.

Prep Time: 15 minutes (plus overnight chilling)

Servings: 2 (easily doubled)

Ingredients:

- ½ cup chia seeds
- 1 cup unsweetened nut milk (almond milk, cashew milk, etc.)
- ¼ cup plain yogurt (Greek yogurt or regular yogurt)
- ¼ cup fresh or frozen berries (blueberries, raspberries, strawberries, etc.)
- 1 tablespoon honey or maple syrup (optional)
- ¼ cup chopped nuts (almonds, walnuts, pecans, etc.)
- ½ teaspoon vanilla extract (optional)

Instructions:

- Whisk together chia seeds, nut milk, yogurt, honey (if using), and vanilla extract (if using) in a medium bowl.
- Stir in the berries (fresh or frozen) and half of the chopped nuts.
- Cover the bowl and refrigerate for at least 4 hours, or ideally overnight, to allow the chia seeds to absorb the liquid and thicken the pudding.
- Before serving, stir in the remaining chopped nuts for added texture.

Storage Tips: The chia seed pudding can be stored in an airtight container in the refrigerator for up to 4 days.

Nutritional Information: (Approximate per serving) Calories: 300, Protein: 8g, Fat: 15g (including healthy fats from nuts and yogurt), Carbohydrates: 25g (including fiber)

Additional Tips:

- Any nut milk of your choice can be used.
- Feel free to experiment with different types of berries and nuts to find your favorite combination.
- For a thicker pudding, use a slightly lower ratio of liquid to chia seeds (3/4 cup nut milk instead of 1 cup).
- You can add a sprinkle of chia seeds or chopped nuts on top for extra decoration before serving.

Baked Apples with Cinnamon and Walnuts

This classic dessert is simple to make and perfect for a cozy night in. Baked apples are naturally sweet and get a flavor boost from warming cinnamon and crunchy walnuts. Plus, it's a great source of fiber and antioxidants, making it a suitable anti-inflammatory dessert option.

Prep Time: 15 minutes

Cook Time: 30-35 minutes

Servings: 2 (easily doubled)

Ingredients:

- 2 large apples (choose a baking variety like Granny Smith, Honeycrisp, or Braeburn)
- 1/4 cup chopped walnuts
- 2 tablespoons chopped pitted dates (optional, for added sweetness)
- 1 tablespoon melted butter
- 1 teaspoon ground cinnamon

- 1/4 teaspoon ground nutmeg (optional)
- Pinch of salt
- 1/4 cup water

Instructions:

- Preheat the oven to 375°F (190°C).
- Wash and core the apples, leaving the bottoms intact to prevent filling from spilling out. You can use an apple corer or a small knife to carefully remove the core.
- Combine chopped walnuts, chopped dates (if using), melted butter, cinnamon, nutmeg (if using), and salt in a small bowl and mix thoroughly.
- Stuff the apple cavities with the walnut mixture.
- Pour water into the bottom of a baking dish to prevent burning. Place the stuffed apples upright in the baking dish.
- Bake for 30-35 minutes, or until the apples are tender and cooked through. A fork should easily pierce through the flesh.
- Let the apples cool slightly before serving.

Storage Tips: Store leftover baked apples in an airtight container in the refrigerator for up to 3 days. However, the texture may soften a little bit.

Nutritional Information: (Approximate per serving) Calories: 300, Protein: 2g, Fat: 15g (including healthy fats from walnuts), Carbohydrates: 40g (including fiber)

Additional Tips:

- You can drizzle the baked apples with a little honey or maple syrup before serving for extra sweetness.
- For a richer flavor, substitute brown sugar for the chopped dates.

- If you don't have walnuts, you can use another type of chopped nut, such as pecans or almonds.
- Serve the baked apples warm with a scoop of vanilla ice cream or whipped cream for an extra decadent treat.

Turmeric Yogurt Parfait with Mango

This vibrant parfait is a refreshing and healthy dessert that's packed with anti-inflammatory benefits. The combination of creamy yogurt, sweet mango, and earthy turmeric creates a delightful taste and texture experience.

Prep Time: 10 minutes

Servings: 1 serving (easily doubled)

Ingredients:

- ½ cup plain Greek yogurt
- ½ mango, peeled and diced
- 1/2 teaspoon ground turmeric
- Pinch of black pepper (enhances turmeric absorption)
- 1 tablespoon chopped nuts or granola (optional, for added crunch)
- Fresh mint leaves (optional, for garnish)

Instructions:

- Whisk together plain Greek yogurt and ground turmeric in a small bowl until well combined.
- In a serving glass or parfait jar, layer half of the yogurt mixture.
- Top the yogurt layer with half of the diced mango.
- Repeat the layers with the remaining yogurt and mango.
- Sprinkle with chopped nuts or granola (if using) for added texture.
- Garnish with a few fresh mint leaves (if using) for a refreshing touch.

Storage Tips: This parfait is best enjoyed fresh. However, if you need to prepare it in advance, you can store it in an airtight container in the refrigerator for up to 24 hours. The texture of the granola or nuts might soften a little bit.

Nutritional Information: (Approximate per serving) Calories: 250, Protein: 15g, Fat: 5g, Carbohydrates: 30g (including fiber)

Additional Tips:

- Both fresh or frozen mango can be used to prepare this recipe. If using frozen mango, thaw it slightly before dicing.
- For a sweeter parfait, drizzle a little honey or maple syrup on top before serving.
- You can substitute other fruits for the mango, such as berries, pineapple, or papaya.
- If you don't have fresh mint leaves, you can use a sprinkle of ground cinnamon for a different flavor profile.

Frozen Yogurt Bark with Berries and Granola

This frozen yogurt bark is a healthy and refreshing treat that's perfect for a hot summer day. It's also a great option for meal prepping healthy snacks. Packed with protein from yogurt and fiber from berries and granola, it's a satisfying and anti-inflammatory dessert option.

Prep Time: 5 minutes

Freeze Time: 3-4 hours (or overnight for best results)

Servings: 4-6 servings (depending on how you break it up)

Ingredients:

- 2 cups plain whole milk yogurt (or Greek yogurt)
- ¼ cup honey or maple syrup

- ½ teaspoon vanilla extract (optional)
- ½ cup fresh or frozen berries of your choice like blueberries, raspberries, strawberries, etc.)
- ¼ cup granola (your favorite kind)

Instructions:

- Arrange a baking sheet with parchment paper.
- Whisk together yogurt, honey or maple syrup, and vanilla extract (if using) in a medium bowl until smooth and well combined.
- Pour the yogurt mixture onto the prepared baking sheet, spreading it into an even layer about ¼ inch thick.
- Sprinkle the berries and granola evenly over the yogurt layer. Gently press them down slightly to ensure they stick.

Freezing:

- Place the baking sheet in the freezer and freeze for at least 3-4 hours, or until the yogurt bark is solid. Ideally, freeze overnight for the best texture.

Cutting and Serving:

- Once frozen, remove the baking sheet from the freezer. Let the bark soften slightly for a few minutes before cutting.
- Break the yogurt bark into pieces of your desired size.

Storage Tips: Frozen yogurt bark can be stored in an airtight container in the freezer for up to 2 weeks.

Nutritional Information: (Approximate per serving, based on a ¼ cup serving size) Calories: 150, Protein: 4g, Fat: 5g, Carbohydrates: 20g (including fiber)

Additional Tips:

- You can use any type of yogurt you prefer, such as vanilla yogurt or flavored yogurt.
- Feel free to experiment with different types of berries and granola to find your favorite combination.
- For a fun twist, drizzle melted dark chocolate or chopped nuts over the yogurt bark before freezing.
- You can add a sprinkle of chia seeds or shredded coconut for extra texture and nutrients.

Poached Pears with Ginger and Spices

This elegant dessert features tender poached pears infused with the warm flavors of ginger and spices. It's a simple yet satisfying treat that's perfect for a special occasion or a cozy night in. Plus, it's a great source of antioxidants and fiber, making it a suitable anti-inflammatory dessert option.

Prep Time: 10 minutes

Cook Time: 35 minutes

Servings: 4 servings

Ingredients:

- 4 ripe but firm pears (such as Bosc or Bartlett)
- 4 cups water
- 1 cup sugar
- 1 cinnamon stick
- 4 whole cloves
- 1 inch knob of fresh ginger, thinly sliced
- 1/4 teaspoon ground cardamom (optional)
- Lemon juice from ½ lemon (optional)

Instructions:

- Combine water, sugar, cinnamon stick, cloves, ginger slices, cardamom (if using), and lemon juice (if using) in a large pot. Bring to a boiling point over medium heat, stirring occasionally until the sugar dissolves.
- While the syrup is heating, peel the pears, leaving the stems intact. You can use a vegetable peeler and carefully leave the bottom part of the pear unpeeled for better presentation.
- Gently lower the pears into the simmering syrup. Make sure the pears are mostly submerged in the liquid. If needed, add a little more water to cover them.
- Reduce heat to low, cover the pot with a lid slightly ajar, and simmer for 20-25 minutes, or until the pears are tender and can be easily pierced with a fork.
- Turn off the heat and let the pears cool slightly in the poaching liquid for at least 15 minutes. This allows them to absorb more flavor.

Serving:

- Transfer the poached pears to serving plates or bowls. Strain the poaching liquid into a serving pitcher or carafe (optional).
- You can serve the pears warm or chilled. Spoon some of the poaching syrup over the pears before serving.

Optional Toppings:

- Vanilla ice cream or a dollop of whipped cream
- A sprinkle of chopped nuts (almonds, walnuts, pistachios)
- A drizzle of honey or maple syrup
- Fresh mint leaves for garnish

Storage Tips: Store leftover poached pears in an airtight container in the poaching liquid in the refrigerator for up to three days.

Nutritional Information: (Approximate per serving) Calories: 300, Protein: 1g, Fat: 0g, Carbohydrates: 75g (including fiber)

Additional Tips:

- You can adjust the amount of sugar in the poaching liquid to your taste preference.
- For a deeper flavor, you can use a variety of spices in the poaching liquid, such as star anise or whole allspice berries.
- If you don't have fresh ginger, you can substitute 1/2 teaspoon of ground ginger. However, fresh ginger will provide a more intense flavor.

Homemade Baked Applesauce

This recipe is a simple and healthy take on applesauce. Baking the apples allows for their natural sweetness to shine through, reducing the need for added sugar. It's a perfect way to use up ripe apples and enjoy a delicious and anti-inflammatory dessert.

Prep Time: 10 minutes

Cook Time: 45-60 minutes

Servings: 4-6 servings (depending on desired consistency)

Ingredients:

- 4-5 apples (tart apples like Granny Smith or a mix of sweet and tart varieties work well)
- 1/4 cup water
- 1/4 teaspoon ground cinnamon
- 1/4 teaspoon ground nutmeg (optional)

- Pinch of salt (optional)

Instructions:

- Preheat the oven to 375°F (190°C).
- Wash and core the apples. You can leave the peels on for extra nutrients and fiber, or peel them if you prefer a smoother texture.
- Cut the apples into wedges or chunks.
- Combine apple pieces, water, cinnamon, nutmeg (if using), and salt (if using) in a large baking dish. Toss to coat the apples evenly.
- Wrap the baking dish with foil or a lid.

Baking:

- Bake for 45-60 minutes, or until the apples are tender and easily mashed with a fork. The baking time may vary depending on the type and ripeness of the apples. Check on them occasionally and stir them halfway through baking to ensure even cooking.

Mashing:

- Once the apples are tender, remove them from the oven. Let them cool slightly.

There are two options for mashing the applesauce:

- ***For a chunky applesauce:*** Use a potato masher or a large fork to mash the apples to your desired consistency. Leave some chunks for a bit of texture.
- ***For a smooth applesauce:*** Transfer the cooked apples to a blender or food processor and puree until smooth. You can add a tablespoon or two of water if needed to achieve a desired consistency.

Serving:

- Serve the applesauce warm or chilled. You can add a sprinkle of ground cinnamon or nutmeg for extra flavor.

Storage Tips: Store leftover applesauce in an airtight container in the refrigerator for up to 5 days. It can also be frozen in freezer-safe containers for up to 3 months.

Nutritional Information: (Approximate per serving, without added sugar) Calories: 100, Protein: 0.5g, Fat: 0.5g, Carbohydrates: 25g (including fiber)

Additional Tips:

- You can add a tablespoon of honey or maple syrup to the apples before baking for a touch of sweetness.
- For a richer flavor, substitute some of the water with apple juice or apple cider.
- Get creative with spices! You can experiment with adding a pinch of ground ginger, cloves, or cardamom to the baking dish for a different flavor profile.

Coconut Milk Chia Pudding with Pineapple

This refreshing and tropical chia pudding is a perfect anti-inflammatory dessert option. Packed with protein and fiber from chia seeds, and the creamy sweetness of coconut milk, it's a healthy and delicious treat. The addition of pineapple chunks provides a burst of vitamins and a delightful tangy counterpoint.

Prep Time: 15 minutes (plus overnight chilling)

Servings: 2 servings (easily doubled)

Ingredients:

- ½ cup chia seeds
- 1 cup unsweetened coconut milk (carton or canned)

- ¼ cup chopped fresh pineapple
- 1 tablespoon honey or maple syrup (optional)
- ½ teaspoon vanilla extract (optional)
- Pinch of salt

Instructions:

- Whisk together chia seeds, coconut milk, honey or maple syrup (if using), vanilla extract (if using), and salt in a medium bowl or jar.
- Stir in the chopped fresh pineapple.
- Cover the bowl or jar and refrigerate for at least 4 hours, or ideally overnight, to allow the chia seeds to absorb the liquid and thicken the pudding.
- Before serving, you can add an extra sprinkle of chopped pineapple or shredded coconut for garnish.

Storage Tips: The chia seed pudding can be stored in an airtight container in the refrigerator for up to 4 days.

Nutritional Information: (Approximate per serving) Calories: 300, Protein: 4g, Fat: 15g (including healthy fats from coconut milk), Carbohydrates: 30g (including fiber)

Additional Tips:

- You can use canned pineapple chunks instead of fresh pineapple, but fresh offers a brighter flavor. If using canned pineapple, drain the excess juice before adding it to the pudding.
- Feel free to experiment with other fruits besides pineapple. Berries, mango, or papaya would also be delicious options.
- For a richer flavor, use full-fat coconut milk instead of unsweetened.
- If you prefer a sweeter pudding, adjust the amount of honey or maple syrup to your taste.

Roasted Sweet Potato with Nut Butter and Berries

This recipe is a simple yet satisfying dessert that's perfect for satisfying a sweet tooth while incorporating anti-inflammatory ingredients. Roasted sweet potatoes provide natural sweetness and complex carbohydrates, while nut butter adds protein and healthy fats. Berries are a rich source of antioxidants and vitamins.

Prep Time: 10 minutes

Cook Time: 40-45 minutes

Servings: 1 serving (easily doubled)

Ingredients:

- 1 medium sweet potato
- 1 tablespoon nut butter (almond butter, peanut butter, cashew butter, etc.)
- ¼ cup fresh berries (blueberries, raspberries, strawberries, etc.)
- 1 tablespoon chopped nuts (almonds, walnuts, pecans, etc.) (optional)
- Pinch of ground cinnamon (optional)
- Pinch of sea salt (optional)

Instructions:

- Preheat the oven to 400°F (200°C).
- Wash and scrub the sweet potato. You can leave the skin on for added nutrients and fiber, or peel it if you prefer a smoother texture.
- Pierce the sweet potato with a fork a few times. This allows steam to escape and helps it cook evenly.
- Arrange the sweet potato on a baking sheet covered with parchment paper.
- Roast the sweet potato for 40-45 minutes, or until tender when pierced with a fork.

Assembly:

- Once the sweet potato is cooked, remove it from the oven and let it cool slightly.
- Cut the sweet potato in half lengthwise or into wedges.
- Spread the chosen nut butter over the cut surface of the sweet potato.
- Top the sweet potato with fresh berries.
- Sprinkle with chopped nuts (if using), ground cinnamon (if using), and a pinch of sea salt (if using) for additional flavor and texture.

Serving Tips:

- This recipe can be enjoyed warm or at room temperature.
- For a richer flavor, drizzle the sweet potato with a teaspoon of honey or maple syrup before adding the toppings.
- Vanilla yogurt or a dollop of whipped cream can be added for an extra decadent treat.

Storage Tips: Store leftover roasted sweet potato in an airtight container in the refrigerator for up to three days. Reheat in the microwave or oven before using again. However, the berries might become slightly softer.

Nutritional Information: (Approximate per serving) Calories: 350, Protein: 4g, Fat: 15g (including healthy fats from nut butter, Carbohydrates: 40g (including fiber)

Additional Tips:

- You can experiment with different types of nut butters and toppings to create your own flavor combinations.
- For a more decadent version, try stuffing the roasted sweet potato with a dollop of mashed ricotta cheese before adding the toppings.

Edamame with Sea Salt

Edamame are young soybeans in their pods, a popular appetizer or snack option. They're a great source of protein and fiber, making them a satisfying and anti-inflammatory choice.

Prep Time: 5 minutes

Cook Time: 5-7 minutes

Servings: 1 serving (easily doubled or tripled)

Ingredients:

- 1 cup frozen shelled edamame
- Water
- Pinch of salt
- Flaky sea salt (for serving)

Instructions:

- Boil a pot of water to a boiling point. Add a pinch of salt (optional) to the boiling water.
- Transfer the frozen edamame to the boiling water.
- Cook the edamame for 5-7 minutes, or according to package instructions, until tender but still bright green.
- Drain the edamame in a colander and rinse briefly with cold water to stop the cooking process.
- Transfer the edamame to a bowl.
- Sprinkle it with flaky sea salt to taste.

Storage Tips: Store leftover cooked edamame in an airtight container in the refrigerator for up to 3 days. However, the texture may become slightly mushy. It's best enjoyed fresh.

Nutritional Information: (Approximate per 1 cup serving) Calories: 180, Protein: 17g, Fat: 8g (including healthy fats), Carbohydrates: 13g (including fiber)

Additional Tips:

- You can buy frozen edamame pre-shelled or in pods. Shelling your own edamame can add a little more prep time, but it can also be a fun activity.
- For a variation, try drizzling the cooked edamame with a little sesame oil or chili oil before adding the sea salt.
- Edamame pods are generally not eaten, but you can discard them after shelling the edamame.

Cucumber Slices with Hummus

This refreshing and light snack is a perfect combination of healthy fats from hummus and hydration from cucumbers. It's simple to make, easy to take on the go, and suitable for individuals with fibromyalgia due to its anti-inflammatory properties.

Prep Time: 5 minutes

Servings: 2-3 servings

Ingredients:

- 1 medium cucumber, sliced into rounds or sticks
- 1 cup hummus (any flavor you prefer)
- Optional toppings: Everything bagel seasoning, sesame seeds, chopped fresh herbs (parsley, mint)

Instructions:

- Wash and dry the cucumber. Slice the cucumber into rounds or sticks, whichever you prefer.
- Arrange the cucumber slices on a plate or serving platter.
- Serve the hummus alongside the cucumber slices for dipping.

Optional Serving Variations:

- Spread a dollop of hummus on each cucumber slice for a more hands-on eating experience.
- For a more flavorful presentation, sprinkle the cucumber slices or hummus with everything bagel seasoning, sesame seeds, or chopped fresh herbs like parsley or mint.

Storage Tips: Store leftover hummus in an airtight container in the refrigerator for up to three days. Sliced cucumber is best enjoyed fresh, but can be stored in an airtight container in the refrigerator for up to a day. However, the texture might become slightly soft.

Nutritional Information: (Approximate per serving with plain hummus and no toppings) Calories: 150, Protein: 4g (from hummus), Fat: 8g (healthy fats from hummus), Carbohydrates: 15g (including fiber from cucumber)

Additional Tips:

- You can choose any flavor of hummus you like, such as roasted red pepper hummus, black bean hummus, or garlic hummus.
- For a more protein-rich snack, pair the cucumber slices with roasted chickpeas or lentil dip instead of hummus.

Apple Slices with Almond Butter

This simple yet satisfying snack combines the natural sweetness of apples with the protein and healthy fats of almond butter. It's a perfect anti-inflammatory snack option due to the fiber content in apples and the anti-inflammatory benefits of almonds.

Prep Time: 5 minutes

Servings: 1 serving (easily doubled)

Ingredients:

- 1 apple (choose a crisp variety like Granny Smith, Pink Lady, or Honeycrisp)
- 2 tablespoons of almond butter or any nut butter of your choice
- Optional toppings: Ground cinnamon, chopped nuts (almonds, walnuts, etc.), sliced banana, raisins

Instructions:

- Wash and dry the apple.
- Slice the apple into thin wedges or rounds.
- Spread almond butter on the apple slices. You can spread it on one side or both sides, depending on your preference.

Optional Serving Variations:

- Sprinkle the apple slices with a pinch of ground cinnamon for extra flavor.
- Top the apple slices with chopped nuts, sliced banana, or raisins for added texture and taste.

Storage Tips: Sliced apples and almond butter are best enjoyed fresh. However, store leftover apple slices in an airtight container in the refrigerator for up to a day, but they may brown slightly. Leftover almond butter can be stored in its original container at room temperature for up to 3 months.

Nutritional Information: (Approximate per serving with 2 tablespoons almond butter) Calories: 300, Protein: 5g (from almond butter), Fat: 13g (including healthy fats from almond butter), Carbohydrates: 35g (including fiber from apple)

Additional Tips:

- You can substitute any nut butter you prefer, such as peanut butter, cashew butter, or sunflower seed butter, for the almond butter.
- If you're concerned about the apple slices browning, you can dip them in a little lemon juice or water with a squeeze of lemon before spreading the almond butter.

Roasted Chickpeas with Turmeric and Spices

These crunchy roasted chickpeas are a protein-packed and flavorful anti-inflammatory snack. Turmeric offers anti-inflammatory benefits, while the spices add a delightful taste dimension.

Prep Time: 15 minutes

Cook Time: 30-35 minutes

Servings: 2-3 servings

Ingredients:

- 1 can (15.5 oz) chickpeas, drained and rinsed
- 1 tablespoon olive oil
- 1 teaspoon ground turmeric
- ½ teaspoon smoked paprika
- ¼ teaspoon ground cumin (optional)
- ¼ teaspoon chili powder (optional)

- Pinch of cayenne pepper (optional, for a kick)
- ½ teaspoon garlic powder
- ¼ teaspoon onion powder
- Pinch of salt
- Black pepper to taste

Instructions:

- Preheat the oven to 375°F (190°C). Arrange baking sheet with parchment paper for easy cleanup.
- Gently toss the drained and rinsed chickpeas with olive oil in a large bowl.
- Add all the spices: turmeric, smoked paprika, cumin (if using), chili powder (if using), cayenne pepper (if using), garlic powder, onion powder, salt, and black pepper.
- Make sure the chickpeas are evenly coated with the spice mixture.
- Spread the chickpeas on the prepared baking sheet in a single layer. For even roasting, ensure not to overcrowd the pan.
- Roast the chickpeas for 30-35 minutes, or until golden brown and crispy. Shake the baking sheet occasionally to ensure even browning.

Serving Suggestions:

- Enjoy the roasted chickpeas warm or at room temperature.
- You can sprinkle them with additional spices like smoked paprika or nutritional yeast for a flavor boost.
- For a more decadent snack, drizzle the roasted chickpeas with a touch of honey or maple syrup before serving.

Storage Tips: Store leftover roasted chickpeas in an airtight container at room temperature for up to 3 days. They can also be stored in an airtight container in the refrigerator for up to a week, but they may lose some crispness.

Nutritional Information: (Approximate per serving) Calories: 200, Protein: 8g, Fat: 5g (including healthy fats), Carbohydrates: 20g (including fiber)

Additional Tips:

- You can experiment with different spice combinations to create your own flavor profiles. Try adding a pinch of ground coriander, ginger, or even a dash of curry powder.
- Roasted chickpeas are a versatile snack and can be enjoyed on their own, added to salads or yogurt parfaits, or used as a topping for soups or bowls.

Bell Pepper Strips with Guacamole

This vibrant and healthy snack is a perfect combination of vitamin C-rich bell peppers and creamy, nutrient-dense guacamole. It's a simple, anti-inflammatory option that's both satisfying and delicious.

Prep Time: 10 minutes

Servings: 1-2 servings

Ingredients:

- 1 bell pepper (red, yellow, orange, or green)
- 1/2 avocado, ripe but firm
- 1 tablespoon chopped red onion (optional)
- 1 tablespoon lime juice
- Pinch of salt
- Black pepper to taste
- Optional toppings: Chopped fresh cilantro, chopped cherry tomatoes

Instructions:

- Wash and dry the bell pepper. Cut the bell pepper into thin strips or slices.
- Mash the avocado with a fork in a bowl until slightly chunky.
- Add the chopped red onion (if using), lime juice, salt, and black pepper to the mashed avocado.
- Stir the guacamole mixture until well combined and the desired consistency is reached.

Serving:

- Arrange the bell pepper strips on a plate or serving platter.
- Serve the guacamole alongside the bell pepper strips for dipping.

Optional Serving Variations:

- Spoon a dollop of guacamole onto each bell pepper strip for a more hands-on eating experience.
- Garnish the guacamole with chopped fresh cilantro or chopped cherry tomatoes for a pop of color and freshness.

Storage Tips: Guacamole is best enjoyed fresh. However, leftover guacamole can be stored in an airtight container in the refrigerator for up to 1 day. To prevent browning, press plastic wrap directly onto the surface of the guacamole to minimize air exposure.

Nutritional Information:(Approximate per serving with red bell pepper and no optional toppings) Calories: 200, Protein: 3g (from avocado), Fat: 15g (including healthy fats from avocado), Carbohydrates: 15g (including fiber from bell pepper)

Additional Tips:

- You are free to use any color bell pepper of your choice. Each color offers slightly different nutrients and flavors.

- If you don't have red onion, you can substitute it with a shallot or green onion for a milder onion flavor.
- Guacamole can also be enjoyed with other dippers like carrot sticks, cucumber slices, or whole-wheat crackers.

Trail Mix with Nuts, Seeds, and Dried Fruit

This customizable trail mix is a perfect anti-inflammatory snack option. It's packed with protein, healthy fats, fiber, and antioxidants from a variety of nuts, seeds, and dried fruits. You can create your own perfect mix to suit your taste and dietary needs.

Prep Time: 10 minutes

Servings: 2-3 servings (depending on portion size)

Ingredients:

- 1 ½ cups raw nuts (almonds, pecans, cashews, peanuts, walnuts, etc.)
- 1 cup raw seeds (sunflower seeds, pumpkin seeds, chia seeds, flaxseeds, etc.)
- 1 cup dried fruit (unsweetened or lightly sweetened raisins, cranberries, cherries, chopped apricots, chopped dates, etc.)
- Optional additions: Dark chocolate chips (antioxidant benefits, choose at least 70% cacao), shredded coconut (healthy fats and fiber), mini pretzels (for a sweet and salty mix)

Instructions:

- Combine all your chosen nuts, seeds, and dried fruits in a large bowl.
- If using chocolate chips, shredded coconut, or mini pretzels, add them to the bowl and mix everything together until well combined.

Storage Tips: Store your trail mix in an airtight container at room temperature for up to a week. However, for optimal freshness, it's recommended to store it in the refrigerator for up to 2 weeks or the freezer for up to 3 months.

Nutritional Information: (Approximate per serving with basic ingredients - nuts, seeds, and dried fruits) Calories: 400, Protein: 10g, Fat: 20g (including healthy fats from nuts and seeds), Carbohydrates: 40g (including fiber from nuts, seeds, and dried fruits)

Additional Tips:

- When choosing nuts, opt for raw or dry roasted varieties with no added salt or unhealthy fats.
- Select unsweetened or lightly sweetened dried fruits to minimize added sugar intake.
- Feel free to experiment with different combinations of nuts, seeds, and dried fruits to create your own favorite trail mix flavor profiles.
- Be mindful of portion sizes, as trail mix can be calorie-dense.
- Hard-Boiled Eggs

Sliced Vegetables with Cottage Cheese

This refreshing and light snack combines the protein and calcium from cottage cheese with the vitamins and fiber from colorful vegetables. It's a simple, customizable, and anti-inflammatory snack option.

Prep Time: 5 minutes

Servings: 1 serving (easily doubled)

Ingredients:

- 1 cup assorted vegetables, sliced into sticks or rounds (choose your favorites - cucumber, bell peppers, carrots, celery, cherry tomatoes, etc.)
- ½ cup low-fat cottage cheese

- Pinch of salt (optional)
- Freshly ground black pepper to taste
- Optional garnishes: Chopped fresh herbs (parsley, chives, dill), everything bagel seasoning

Instructions:

- Wash and dry your chosen vegetables. For easy dipping, slice them into sticks or rounds.
- Combine the cottage cheese with a pinch of salt (if using) and freshly ground black pepper in a bowl.
- Arrange the sliced vegetables on a plate or serving platter.
- Serve the cottage cheese dip alongside the vegetables for dipping.

Optional Serving Variations:

- Spoon a dollop of cottage cheese onto each vegetable slice for a more hands-on eating experience.
- Sprinkle the cottage cheese or vegetables with chopped fresh herbs like parsley, chives, or dill for an extra flavor boost.
- Add a sprinkle of everything bagel seasoning to the cottage cheese or vegetables for a savory and flavorful twist.

Storage Tips: Store leftover sliced vegetables in an airtight container in the refrigerator for up to a day, but they may lose some crispness. Store leftover cottage cheese in its original container in the refrigerator for up to 5 days.

Nutritional Information: (Approximate per serving with low-fat cottage cheese and no optional garnishes) Calories: 150, Protein: 15g (from cottage cheese), Fat: 3g (from cottage cheese), Carbohydrates: 15g (including fiber from vegetables)

Additional Tips:

- You can choose a variety of colorful vegetables to add different vitamins and minerals to your snack.
- For a thicker dip, you can blend or mash some of the cottage cheese to create a smoother consistency.
- If you prefer a creamier dip, add a tablespoon of plain Greek yogurt to the cottage cheese.

Rice Cakes with Sliced Avocado and Smoked Salmon

This is a delicious and satisfying snack that perfectly combines the benefits of complex carbohydrates from rice cakes with healthy fats and protein from avocado and smoked salmon. It's a great anti-inflammatory option due to the omega-3 fatty acids found in smoked salmon.

Prep Time: 5 minutes

Servings: 1 serving (easily doubled)

Ingredients:

- 2 plain rice cakes
- 1/2 ripe avocado, sliced
- 2-3 slices smoked salmon
- Squeeze of lemon juice (optional)
- Pinch of salt and freshly ground black pepper (optional)

Instructions:

- Wash and dry the avocado. Slice the avocado into thin slices.
- Squeeze a little lemon juice on the avocado slices if desired, to prevent browning.
- Place the rice cakes on a plate.

Assembly:

- Arrange the avocado slices on top of the rice cakes.

- Top the avocado slices with smoked salmon.

Optional Seasoning:

- Season with a pinch of salt and freshly ground black pepper to taste.

Serving Tips:

- You can add a sprinkle of everything bagel seasoning or chopped fresh herbs like dill for an extra flavor boost.
- For a creamier option, spread a thin layer of mashed avocado on the rice cakes before adding the smoked salmon.

Storage Tips: This snack is best enjoyed fresh as the avocado can brown over time. Store leftover smoked salmon in an airtight container in the refrigerator for up to three days. Store leftover rice cakes in their original packaging at room temperature for up to a week.

Nutritional Information: (Approximate per serving) Calories: 300, Protein: 8g (from smoked salmon), Fat: 15g (including healthy fats from avocado and smoked salmon), Carbohydrates: 30g (including fiber from rice cakes)

Additional Tips:

- You can choose brown rice cakes for added fiber content.
- If you don't have smoked salmon, other smoked fish options like mackerel or trout can be used.

Conclusion

As we reach the final chapter of this journey, let's revisit the profound impact an anti-inflammatory diet can have on managing fibromyalgia. Chronic inflammation is now understood to play a significant role in fibromyalgia symptoms, including pain, fatigue, and sleep disturbances. By incorporating anti-inflammatory foods and minimizing pro-inflammatory ones, you've taken a crucial step towards reclaiming your well-being.

This book has equipped you with the knowledge to make informed choices about the fuel you put into your body. You've learned about the power of nutrient-rich fruits, vegetables, whole grains, and healthy fats to reduce inflammation and support your overall health. Lifestyle modification is another game changer in managing and treating the symptoms of fibromyalgia.

Maintaining a healthy lifestyle can be challenging, especially when dealing with chronic pain. Here are some tips you will need to stay motivated:

Celebrate your victories: Acknowledge even small improvements in your symptoms or energy levels.

Focus on progress, not perfection: There will be slip-ups. Don't let them discourage your journey. Get it right with your next meal.

Find an accountability partner: Share your journey with a friend or family member who can offer support and encouragement.

Make healthy eating enjoyable: Experiment with recipes, explore new cuisines, and discover the delicious possibilities of anti-inflammatory cooking.

Cook in bulk: Prepare healthy meals on the weekends to save time and avoid unhealthy temptations during busy weekdays.

This book has provided you with the foundation, but your anti-inflammatory journey doesn't end here. The world of anti-inflammatory cuisine is vast and exciting. Don't be scared about experimenting with different flavors and ingredients. Explore herbs and spices that not only add zest but also boast anti-inflammatory properties. Embrace diverse cooking styles like Mediterranean, Indian, or Thai, all known for their incorporation of anti-inflammatory ingredients. Remember, a healthy diet is not about deprivation; it's about abundance. It's about nourishing your body with delicious and beneficial foods that empower you to manage your fibromyalgia and live a vibrant life. As you continue on this path, you'll not only discover a wealth of culinary delights but also experience a renewed sense of well-being and vitality.

Finally, managing fibromyalgia can be a daily challenge, but you are not alone. By embracing an anti-inflammatory diet and making healthy choices, you are taking control of your health and paving the way for a brighter future. Remember, small changes can create significant improvements. With dedication and a spirit of exploration, you can turn anti-inflammatory eating into a sustainable lifestyle that supports you on your journey towards a life filled with less pain and more vibrancy.